Mastering the Health Continuum

8 Daily Practices to Boost Energy, Optimize Health, and Age Gracefully

Dr. Nancy Miggins

Mastering the Health Continuum / Nancy Miggins

ISBN: 978-1-7331299-0-9

It's Time to Transform Your Health

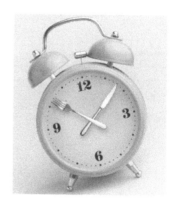

Get Your FREE Planner

Read This First

I have put together an 8 Daily Practices Planner to enhance your Mastering the Health Continuum experience. It includes templates and resources for you to use for tracking your metrics, identifying your key priority, planning your meals and scheduling your daily practices.

Every success is founded in good habits and mastering your health is no different. Download your FREE planner at **www.drnancymiggins.com/8-practices-planner**

For Kenna

"The best time to plant a tree was 20 years ago.
The second-best time is now."

—Chinese Proverb

Contents

Introduction

"Your body is your most priceless possession.
Take Care of it."

—Jack Lalane

We are all aging. From conception to birth, we all go through a cycle of growth and degeneration. Thus, aging and death are inevitable. No one lives this life forever.

Throughout our lives, we earn wrinkles, gray hair, baldness and shriveled bodies. We bear the marks and scars of battles won and lost during a life well lived. As our bodies fade, our wisdom grows and we become more interesting, adding more dimension to our character. Beauty and vitality are entrenched below our skin, and they continue to radiate through our deteriorating exterior. *Mastering The Health Continuum* goes beyond aesthetic vanity and instead focuses on optimizing you on the inside to fuel the flame of your vitality so your inner beauty will long outlive your outer beauty.

With the abundance of information available at your fingertips—Google, Facebook, Amazon, Instagram, You Tube, and Pinterest—you have endless options for diets, exercise, miracle drinks, recipes, fads, and gimmicks. Websites, blogs, and even celebrities have dedicated their time and energy to providing innovative solutions for your health. But how do you know which solutions are true? Not everything "out there" is false or misleading; however, it is difficult to wade through all of that information and determine what is real, true, and most importantly, wise.

The age of selfies and living out loud online has caused an epidemic of comparison, as opposed to inspiration, that is eroding our self-confidence and self-love. Our unique minds, bodies, and life experiences make us interesting and beautiful.

Yet if an online post shows pictures of a beautiful young woman who has lost fifteen pounds in two weeks drinking a special concoction, how can you feel good about yourself? You think you are eating a good diet and exercising appropriately, but you still do not look like her. We are inundated with pressure and noise constantly reminding us of the unrealistic expectations we have set around beauty, health, healing, and aging for that matter. It is an illusion with an impossible immediacy to achieve.

Those photos do not show that same young woman three months or even two years later. They don't show the impact that her myopic actions have had on her body. Yes, she may look great on her wedding day or for that cruise, but every action has a consequence. Some consequences are worse than others. For example, ever-popular fad dieting has detrimental effects on your thyroid, kidneys, liver, mitochondria, and even your gut health, brain function, and fertility.

There is no "one-size-fits-all" answer. Bio-individuality is a key consideration when determining the most appropriate plan or program to follow to achieve your health goals.

Over the years, many of my patients have appreciated my approach to helping them develop an appropriate health strategy based on their unique bio-individuality. They say it is the first time they have worked with a practitioner and have felt heard, not shamed or judged.

Keeping your bio-individuality in mind, you need to know where you are right now on the health continuum, what health challenges you are experiencing, and your end goal. You can then efficiently and intelligently sift through your options, determining what will bring you closer to or further away from your goal.

Ultimately, what matters most is how you feel about yourself and the progress you make toward your goals. This journey is about you compared to you. You are not in a race against anyone else. Your starting point, health challenges, and commitment to achieving your goals determine your results.

Many things can get in the way of our success. The most common is fear. Whether or not it is fear of failure, fear of success, fear of inability, fear of disappointment, fear of criticism and judgement, fear of the unknown, or all of the above, fear is a major paralyzing force in our lives.

What if fear is your opportunity? We all know that eliminating fear is a losing battle. Embrace it. Lean into it. Be honest with yourself. Let your fears fuel and motivate your passions and actions.

I really hate to be the one to tell you this, but no one is going to show up to rescue you or do this work for you. Hopefully, you are not expecting that. You need to be the one to make the decision and take action to make your health the priority.

While you can come up with a variety of excuses to not make it a priority, you need to decide to not give in to your fears or excuses—no one can do it for you. We all feel that we have an overabundance of demands placed on us. Work, family, social obligations, and philanthropy efforts all tend to take precedence over our individual needs. We put off eating intentional and delicious food in favor of convenience. We put off the exercise that we know we need in favor of the unexpected requests from the people we love or because we are just too damn tired. We don't want to disappoint or inconvenience those people in our lives that matter to us. In general, we procrastinate and lower the priority of the activities that will keep us healthy and vibrant.

In that light, I want to remind you that flight attendants instruct you to put your own oxygen mask on first before helping others because if you don't take care of yourself first, you will not be in a position to help others. The same applies to your health.

Making health your top priority serves two purposes:

1. It positions you to be able to care for others.

2. It acts as an example for everyone else in your life, making a commitment to healthy habits contagious.

This book can help you with your commitment. I do not claim to have all of the answers and this is not a silver bullet, but I hope this book can answer some of your questions, raise other questions for you, and inspire you to take ownership of your health journey.

The daily practices outlined in this book can help you achieve a strong foundation of health, optimize your body's physiology, and increase your vitality. You may not lose weight immediately. You may not experience less pain or more energy right away. You may not feel any different in the short term. And for some of you, you may even feel worse, at least for a while.

Ultimately, the results you achieve are a direct consequence of your choices and actions. Your spirit resides in the only body it will have during this life. You deserve to love and nurture yourself. And if you don't, who will? It all starts with you.

Order out of Chaos

I am a very process-oriented person. Systems and processes are the basis of efficiency. They provide the foundation and framework for predictable outcomes and results.

To create a functional, reproducible, and sustainable system, one must start with the most basic elements. I used this same process to develop this book.

I combined my advanced education, patient practice experience, business operation experience, and years of reading and researching solutions for patients, friends, and family. I then broke it all down into the most elemental pieces and built from that a system of daily practices. Out of all of the chaos of information, I created order.

I focused in on health strategies that do not require special equipment, supplements, gym membership, or a personal trainer. All of these practices can be facilitated wherever you are, whether or not you are at home, your office, or a hotel room. I did my best to remove many of the obstacles that prevent people from taking action in the short term and staying the course for a lifetime.

These practices are all tried and true strategies that I have used personally and recommended to patients. While there are many options "out there," these are solid and timeless approaches. You may recognize some or all of them. You may even have tried some or all of them in the past.

Even if you have tried some of these elements independently before and not realized the results you were hoping for, I sure hope you love yourself enough to try one more time under the guidance of this system. You have nothing to lose and everything to gain. The ideal components practiced in combination can consistently bring about miraculous results.

Magic happens when you are at the right place at the right time. I want to thank you in advance for being intrigued and trusting me enough to read this book and consider my approach.

I have included some science in the form of anatomy and physiology to help provide the nitty gritty "why" for these practices. But I have intentionally attempted to keep the information and practices as simple as possible so that they are understandable, doable, and sustainable for the long haul.

The Eight Daily Practices

On one hand, each of the eight daily practices are independent of each other. On the other, they are intimately interwoven, connected, and synergistic. Each practice builds on the next.

The eight practices are connected. If you aren't getting adequate sleep, this will impact your overall results even if you are diligent in your practice of the other seven. Optimal exercise with a poor diet or inadequate hydration can have deleterious health consequences. Your ability to create health, or create disease for that matter, is determined by how well you perform all eight practices.

Learning this system of daily practices is not rigid in the sense that they need to occur in any particular order. However, I have organized them in a way which I feel will provide you with the best result.

Part three of the book pulls it all together and provides suggestions on how to integrate these practices into your day. I can't stress enough that consistency is key to maximizing the results.

I suggest that you read, adopt, and master each practice before moving on to the next one. This will help you avoid "system overload," which could cause you to toss this book aside, feeling defeated before you even start.

In order to master each practice, take each step at a time. Little steps in a direction can often lead to big results. Just keep taking little steps as small achievements build confidence.

The amount of time required for each step depends on you—not on how much time you put in, but more about where you are starting from. For instance, if you already sleep at least eight hours every night like a baby, then the Zzzz practice may not take any time at all to master as opposed to a sleep-challenged person who may takes weeks to finally find peace and rest. Likewise, if you are in stellar fitness and enjoy an optimal body weight and Body Mass Index (BMI), then the movement practice may be an easy transition. But if you are fairly deconditioned, it may take you months to develop the confidence, strength, and flexibility needed to master the movement practice.

This does not mean that you won't find value in that particular information, or in the information contained throughout the rest of the book. Hopefully, my explanations of the "why" will help to deepen your commitment to the practices outlined.

Be gentle with yourself. Love yourself. Be patient and trust the process.

Measure

Knowing your starting point is important information. It is nearly impossible to map how to get to your desired destination without first knowing where you are.

I experienced this frustration firsthand years ago when I was at a women's leadership training. The facilitator broke us into groups of five and gave us a map, a compass, and key coordinates.

Given we were all intelligent, professional women, we were not intimidated by this exercise—until the instructions were given. We had five minutes to discuss our plan and come to consensus. After five minutes we were to be "on silence," move toward our destination, and no longer discuss our plan. The entire group had to move together. So faster moving people had to move slower so that the slower moving people could keep up.

If at any point the group fell out of consensus, that is if any one person questioned the direction or course, we were instructed to stop. We could speak again to gain consensus, but as soon as we moved in a direction we were "on silence" again.

Many of the groups were quick to move even if they were moving in the wrong direction. They strategized that moving in any direction was better than standing still.

Our group was different. We immediately recognized that if we didn't identify our starting point, we really couldn't determine how to get to the destination or the most efficient route. In our group a woman needed a cane to assist her walking. We were in foothills with very hilly terrain and would need to travel cross-country without a road or trail. Considering our teammate's disability, we felt it would benefit us, and her, to spend more time planning so we could avoid unnecessary trekking for our teammate. If she couldn't finish the exercise, none of us would.

Even though all of the other teams had disappeared from view, we stayed true to our strategy. It only took an extra ten minutes to map out a course that we felt confident would take us to the finish line. We plotted the shortest route to minimize the burden on our teammate.

It was difficult to stay on track because of the distractions from the other teams; we could see them heading in different directions and would periodically stop to discuss if we needed to adjust our plan. Ultimately, by staying true to our well-planned strategy and monitoring our progress, we were the first team to arrive at the destination in spite of our slow walking and frequent stops to allow our teammate to rest. We walked the shortest distance compared to all the other teams.

As you can see, you must know your starting point. Do not be deterred by the distraction and activity of anyone else. Your journey and your strategy are unique to you.

There are metrics associated with each practice. Measuring and documenting your baselines and your daily progress will help keep you on track even when your motivation and confidence might be challenged. Tracking helps to keep you accountable.

Please do not feel ashamed if you can't meet a particular goal. Remember, this is a process, not a destination. The goals outlined are just a target. They are an ideal designed to keep you moving in the right direction.

By tracking your results, you will be able to easily visualize your progress, even if you are not "feeling" any changes, yet. Change and healing will happen on the cellular level before you notice any physical shift in symptoms.

You can download a daily tracking sheet from my website at www.drnancymiggins.com. Or you can create your own. I suggest putting together a binder to keep the results you compile over time.

I am both humbled and honored to be part of your journey.

Part 1: A New Paradigm

"The power that made the body heals the body."

— BJ Palmer

Health Continuum

We are on a health continuum from conception to death. Some might argue that our health is affected and influenced by the behavior and lifestyle choices of our parents prior to conception. This reinforces the idea that health, and disease for that matter, are not stagnant. Health is not a destination, but rather a process strongly influenced by the choices you make (or choices that your parents made prior to you) in regard to diet and lifestyle.

Disease is often a more tangible and measurable state of being. A profile of symptoms leads to a diagnosis, labeling your current state and making it much easier for you to locate yourself on the health continuum. Health, on the other hand, is more elusive. It is more like that carrot being dangled out in front of you that you can never quite reach or grasp.

OPTIMAL HEALTH

- Energy
- Mental resilience
- Physical resilience
- Alkaline PH
- Quality sleep

Comfort Zone

- Inconsistent nutrition
- Sporadic exercise
- Inconsistent energy

- Fatigue
- Weight gain
- High stress
- Poor sleep
- Health issues
- Medication

DISEASE

Health

Health is more than the absence of disease or symptoms. It is a state of optimal physical and emotional well-being. Optimal, not normal. Normal ranges have more significance when it comes to identifying disease, not health. Your unique makeup and where you fall on the health continuum determine what that optimum is for you.

Conventional wisdom has often left people powerless to combat disease when they are diagnosed since many believe that our genes determine our fate and there is nothing that we can do to change that. While our genetics do play a role, our genetic predisposition or susceptibility does not equate to genetic realization. This is great news! This means that even if we have a family prevalence of heart disease, diabetes, or cancer, disease is not our destiny.

Your day-to-day diet and lifestyle choices influence your genes. These choices have a direct effect on your well-being and the welfare of future generations. The science behind this, epigenetics, is proving that we have control over and responsibility for the integrity of our genes.

You are born with a genetic code that helps determine your physical traits, like hair, eye, and skin color, as well as how your body functions on the inside. Genes, which are made up of DNA, are located on the chromosomes within the nucleus of each of your cells. However, they are not stagnant as they are in a constant state of flux, being "turned on" and "turned off" continually in response to changes in your internal and external environment. Surprisingly, your genetic code may only play as much as 20 percent in predetermining your health. Lifestyle and environment, through the activation, de-activation, and damage of genes determine as much as 80 percent of health and healing potential. That gives you an extraordinary amount of control over your vitality and health destiny.

Designed to be very agile, your body adapts and compensates over time in response to dietary choices, exercise regimes, and environmental influences as it strives to maintain optimal functioning. Your genes are being activated and deactivated as a result of these life choices. Under ideal circumstances, you can gracefully respond to the onslaught of stressors that you are exposed to on a moment-to-moment basis. More often than not, however, circumstances are not ideal, and the body builds itself sick.

Disease begins as dis-ease and stress is at the root of this dysfunction. When the subtle signs and symptoms of imbalance are ignored, or when the inborn stress response becomes chronic, the body has to go to greater measures to try to neutralize the insult or interference. This pushes us along the disease continuum toward death even though more pronounced symptoms and full-blown disease can often take ten–twenty years or more to develop as the body becomes more and more out of alignment and unable to function as intended.

In my experience the vast majority of people are not aware of the health continuum. People do not even consider that they are in a lifetime battle to continually fight against all disease. People want a quick fix because they think their dysfunction is new. But when they don't find that quick fix, they move on with their lives. It is not uncommon to be fairly far down the disease continuum before experiencing enough "pain" to take action and seek resolve. Too often people can have so much deterioration that they do not have enough time left to turn things around and get the pendulum swinging in the right direction to achieve health and improve their quality of life.

This pain might be experienced as physical pain, such as joint pain or muscle aches, and is often associated with a diminishing quality of life. They no longer have the stamina to play golf or tennis, or they struggle to get down on the floor to play with their grandkids, and then struggle even more to get back up. They no longer enjoy sex with their partner due to chronic fatigue and sleep deprivation.

Normal daily activities require more energy and often result in frequent minor injuries.

Your pain does not need to be a complex physical issue, like fibromyalgia or neuropathy, to be considered important. Again, do not judge yourself against others. Your diminishing ability to get into and out of your car, care for yourself and your property, or enjoy your hobbies can result in devastating pain. Feeling shame or guilt about the importance or severity of your "dis-ease" only compounds the problem. Someone else in the world will always be worse off than you, but this does not negate your pain and suffering. Comparing yourself to others will not serve you or your loved ones today or in your pursuit of vitality and a healthy life in the future. When you compare you to you, it creates an environment where you can feel empowered to take control over your lifestyle choices and actions.

Every person's body matters, and because of bio-individuality, it is often a unique combination of factors that inspires a person to seek a solution. I had a patient, a sweet, spunky seventy-five-year-old woman, come to see me for back pain. She was very concerned about her diminishing ability to be the caretaker for her husband who had recently gone blind. I listened to her talk about her life and her goals, and it became very clear to me that her motivation and desire to be more functional was selfless. Sure, she wanted a reduction in her pain, but what she really wanted was to be able to bend over and pick up her 17 lb. cat and lift it up onto her husband's lap.

Because he was blind, he could no longer interact with his beloved cat as he had done for ten years. This sweet woman knew that when her husband had the cat on his lap, he was less distressed and disoriented.

The "why" behind health goals often stems from quality of life. The journey may be as simple as striving to lift a cat or as complex as reversing diabetes. My patient was very clear on her motivation to eliminate her back pain and increase her strength and function. She was devoted to her husband and providing him with a good quality of life, in spite of his blindness. Being clear on the "why" and staying focused on that goal carries you through the peaks and valleys of rebuilding your health.

Our world is fast-paced, and we have come to expect immediate gratification. That is not how health (or your body) works. Just as it takes years and often decades to build disease, it takes time to rebuild health. There is no magic pill or potion that will cure you. Only you can cure you.

The Science Behind
How Our Body Works

Now comes the nitty gritty science part that I referred to earlier. I understand that not everyone is interested in science or biology, let alone nerding out over human anatomy and physiology. If you are reading this book, however, you are most likely interested in your health.

Understanding the key elements behind how your body works will help to remove the fear of the unknown and give you more confidence to reclaim control over your health. Knowledge is power. I promise I will not get too deep. The following topics will help you to understand how the body builds itself healthy and why it builds itself sick.

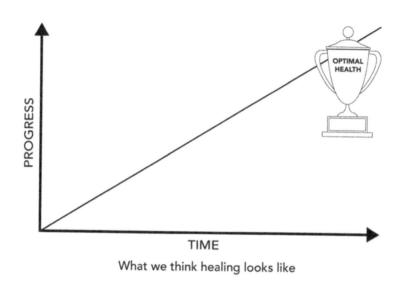

What we think healing looks like

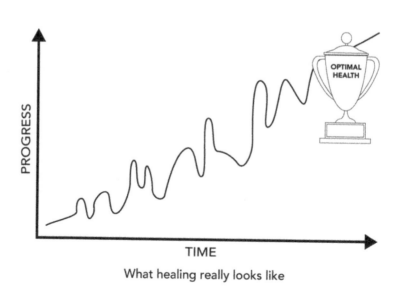

What healing really looks like

The Miracle of Our Innate Intelligence

We are born with an innate, or inborn, intelligence. The body has the ability to heal itself of every disease known to man through this intelligence.

Innate intelligence works through the brain and nervous system to control and coordinate all of the functions of the body. This keeps our heart beating, without interruption or conscious thought. Our heart pumps two gallons of blood per minute throughout the sixty thousand miles of blood vessels in our body. Every blood cell makes a complete tour throughout the body every twenty–sixty seconds. And all of this happens without any conscious thought.

Concurrently, every single second about a hundred thousand chemical reactions take place in every single one of your approximately one trillion cells that make up your body. In the same second, millions of your cells died. You don't have to think about how to get rid of those dead cells or how to coordinate the energy and processes required to create a million new cells to replace them.

Right now, your body is digesting food, filtering blood through the kidneys to produce urine, exchanging oxygen and carbon dioxide in the lungs, and manufacturing a plethora of chemicals that enhance or inhibit every function in your body. Your innate intelligence is constantly scanning the more than 3 billion DNA sequences that comprise the genes located in every one of your cells looking for damage and mutations. On top of that, your body is fighting bacteria and viruses without you even knowing you are under attack, memorizing these onslaughts so the immune system can be better prepared and more efficient the next time it is faced with an invasion, and your mitochondria are constantly producing the energy you need to function.

You are a miracle. There is no one else like you on the planet and there never will be. It all started when two "half cells" came together, a sperm and an egg. Each cell contributed half of your chromosomes and genetic code. In the split second of their union, they created you and established your unique DNA makeup.

But the miracle does not stop here. Upon the union of the sperm and egg, a spark of life stimulates your cells and they start to divide. At first two become four, four become eight, and so on. But on day fifteen, innate wisdom starts to differentiate and organize the cells, forming a primitive streak. This first sign of differentiation, or specialization, is your spinal cord.

As the cells continue to multiply and specialize, the brain is formed at the top of the primitive streak and the nerves grow out bilaterally at precise intervals along its length. Then the individual organs form at the end of the appropriate nerves. The skull, vertebra, and ribs form around the delicate brain, spinal cord, and vital organs to protect them.

And so, the miracle goes, and in nine months you have grown from two "half cells" to 1 trillion cells that all work in unison performing their specific purpose. Your innate intelligence continues to regenerate that life, regulate the incredible number of processes, and maintain order among all of the cells, tissues, organs, and systems of the body. This power that made the body is the power that maintains and heals the body.

I call your attention to the details of how we come to be to remind you that you are truly a miracle. Just think about how many millions of cell divisions occur during the creation of you. In spite of all of the opportunities for error, you are perfect. Elegantly, perfectly imperfect. Each baby born is a unique and awe-inspiring miracle.

The Nervous System Controls Everything

Your nervous system works to ensure the survival of the miracle that is you. The nervous system as a whole activates, controls, and coordinates all bodily functions, integrating the immense complexities of our cells into harmony. It regulates cardiovascular, digestive, immune, endocrine, musculoskeletal, reproductive, and elimination systems.

All day long, day in and day out, the brain, spinal cord, and nerves carry chemical and physical messages to every part of the body. The cells and tissues of the body likewise send communication back to the brain. If this two-way communication between the brain and body happens without any interference, then the body functions as it should by design, and you continue to build health and a healthy body.

Also, by design, the skull and vertebrae work to encase and protect the delicate and vital components of the nervous system. Yet we expose our bodies to an abundance of physical, chemical, and emotional stress and trauma daily, and this certainly takes its toll over the span of our lives. This stress and trauma can cause the bones of the skull and spine to shift out of alignment in an effort to adapt and compensate to preserve maximum function. The subtle shifting of these bony structures can put pressure on the nervous system, causing interference in its ability to communicate clearly and efficiently.

I would often describe this communication loop to patients as the "safety pin cycle." When the brain-body communication pathway is interrupted, it results in a disruption of normal cell, organ, and tissue function. The longer this nerve interference exists, the more damage that can occur to both the nervous system and the organs and tissues it supplies. It can also limit the body's ability to effectively detoxify, properly repair and replace damaged cells, and effectively mount an immune response, and it compromises other critical life-sustaining functions. This is how your body ultimately builds itself sick.

We are more familiar with the concepts of heart health or gut health. But without the nervous system, there would be no life.

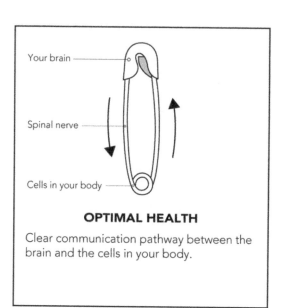

OPTIMAL HEALTH

Clear communication pathway between the brain and the cells in your body.

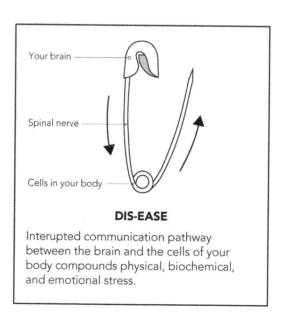

DIS-EASE

Interupted communication pathway between the brain and the cells of your body compounds physical, biochemical, and emotional stress.

The Central Nervous System

Without getting too specific, the nervous system consists of several key components. The **central nervous system** is comprised of the brain and spinal cord. It is generally accepted that the brain has three evolutionary levels:

Hindbrain: Brainstem and Cerebellum
The brainstem is responsible for basic life functions, including maintenance and control of heart rate and breathing. It also regulates sleep and wakefulness.

The cerebellum is responsible for balance, coordination, proprioception, and the execution of controlled movements.

Midbrain: Limbic System
Adjusts our internal state to compensate for changes in our environment. Controls and maintains body temperature, blood pressure, digestion, blood sugar levels, and hormone levels.

Responsible for fight, flee, feed, and fornicate responses.

Forebrain:
Responsible for our ability to think and reason, be aware and creative, and communicate verbally.

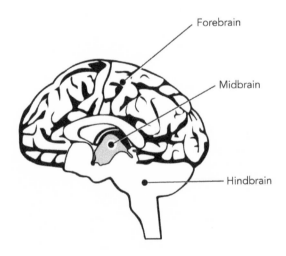

The Peripheral Nervous System

The **peripheral nervous system** includes all of the nerves outside of the brain and spinal cord. These nerves carry impulses from tissues and organs to and from the spinal cord.

The Autonomic Nervous System

The **autonomic nervous system** resides in both the central and peripheral nervous systems with the midbrain playing a crucial governing role. This is the body's self-regulating control system. It regulates body temperature, blood sugar levels, respiratory rates and pulse. The autonomic nervous system plays a key role in regulating and maintaining homeostasis.

The autonomic nervous system has two parts: the sympathetic and parasympathetic. The **sympathetic nervous system** prepares the body for fight or flee. It biochemically alters the body to increase the chance of survival. The **parasympathetic nervous system** works to restore and conserve energy and resources, influencing a rest and rejuvenate response throughout the body.

PARASYMPATHETIC DIVISION
"rest and digest"

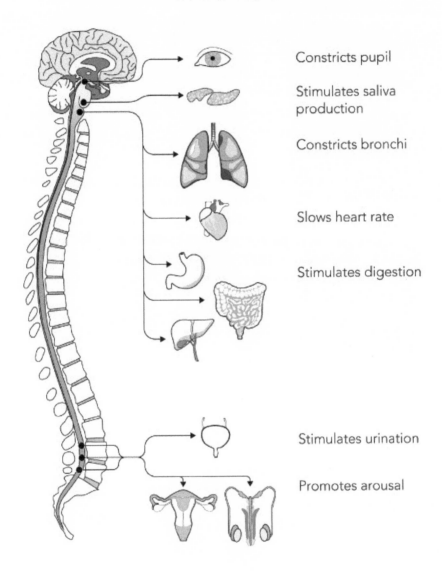

Constricts pupil

Stimulates saliva production

Constricts bronchi

Slows heart rate

Stimulates digestion

Stimulates urination

Promotes arousal

SYMPATHETIC DIVISION
"fight or flight"

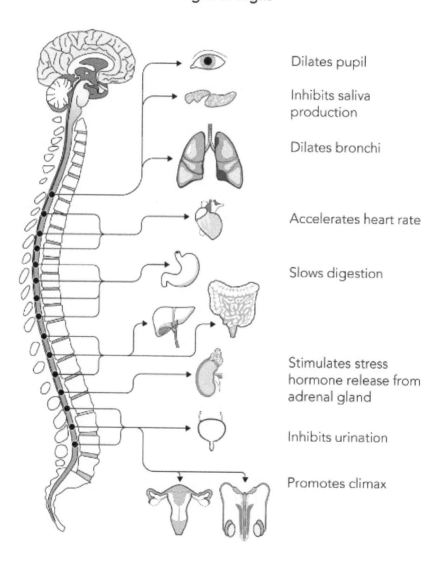

Dilates pupil

Inhibits saliva production

Dilates bronchi

Accelerates heart rate

Slows digestion

Stimulates stress hormone release from adrenal gland

Inhibits urination

Promotes climax

The Mind

As if the brain and nervous system were not complicated enough already, psychoneuroimmunology has demonstrated a link between mind and body. Every thought produces a biochemical reaction in the brain. This results in the brain releasing chemical signals that are sent out into the body. Ultimately, your body feels the way your brain was just thinking.

This is so powerful. When you think happy, positive thoughts your brain manufactures chemicals that make you feel inspired. It works the same way with negative thoughts too, so beware. Your thoughts create your reality. We will talk more about this in practice 8.

Mitochondria: The Body's Powerplant

It takes energy to run our brain and bodily functions and to heal and repair. Our mitochondria are tiny organelles located in almost every cell of the body. They generate all of the energy required by the brain and body to function properly and efficiently. Thus, the health of your mitochondria largely determines the degree of health you enjoy and the rate at which you age.

In fact, because your mitochondria play such an important role in determining your health potential, I am going to share a lot of detail in this section. Hang in there; this is important.

If you can remember back to high school biology, you learned about the Krebs Cycle and the electron transport chain. These are key physiologic processes in the production of energy by your mitochondria.

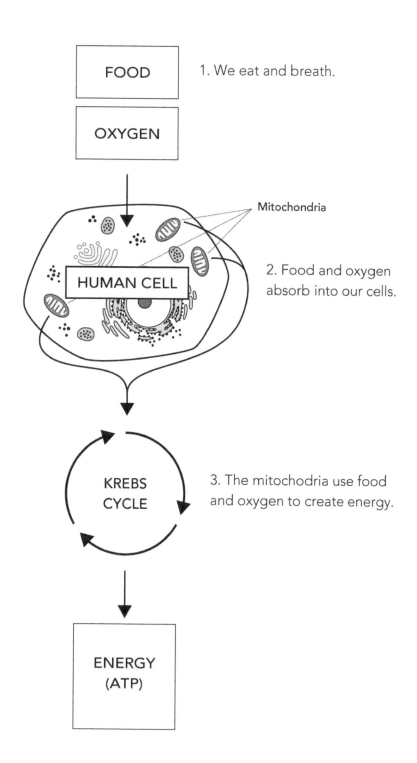

FOOD

OXYGEN

1. We eat and breath.

Mitochondria

HUMAN CELL

2. Food and oxygen absorb into our cells.

KREBS CYCLE

3. The mitochodria use food and oxygen to create energy.

ENERGY (ATP)

Basically, mitochondria use water and oxygen to convert glucose and fatty acids into adenosine triphosphate (ATP), the universal power source in your body. Natural by-products of this manufacturing process are called reactive oxygen species (ROS), a form of free radical. When your body has ample levels of the vital nutrients it needs to operate and maintain balance, it has enough antioxidants available to neutralize the ROS.

ROS are a normal by-product of energy production. Mitochondria are directly exposed to high levels of ROS, making them particularly vulnerable to mitochondrial DNA mutations. These mutations not only interfere with the mitochondria's normal operating procedures and compromise the efficiency in energy production, they also can lead to chronic inflammation, oxidative stress, and cancer. Mitochondrial dysfunction accelerates the aging process.

Thus, you must protect your mitochondria from elements that can inhibit performance and cause damage to their DNA. Many mitochondrial stressors can impair function and promote DNA mutations and damage, including chemicals in the environment, blue light that is emitted from LED bulbs and technology screens, breakdown products of the food we eat, over the counter and prescription drugs used in clinical therapies, and radiation from sunlight or medical procedures. Smoking cigarettes, using recreational drugs, and drinking alcohol can also have a negative impact on mitochondria and their DNA.

The cells in your body cannot store large amounts of ATP for future use. Mitochondria, therefore, have to produce what is needed, moment to moment. By connecting the dots, you can see that dysfunction of these power houses has consequences locally within the cell as well as systemically throughout our body.

Mitochondria have evolved multiple systems of quality control to ensure that the requisite number of functional mitochondria are present to meet the energy demands of the cell in which they are located. This delicate balance is called mitochondrial homeostasis. Our innate intelligence manages this population control. It is so fascinating that all of this fine-tuning takes place without our awareness. Under nutrient-rich conditions, damaged and superfluous mitochondria are selectively weaned to maintain mitochondrial homeostasis. This process is called mitophagy.

The brain and nervous system are particularly vulnerable to mitochondrial dysfunction, mostly since they depend heavily on high energy. For this reason our brain cells have a high concentration of mitochondria. The accurate and proper degradation of dysfunctional mitochondria by mitophagy is essential for maintaining control over mitochondrial quality and quantity in neurons. Even a minor shift in energy production can have a noticeable effect on your brain and cognition.

Autophagy

In addition to having its own power plant, your body also has an inborn cleaning mechanism: autophagy, which means self-eating. This process is part of an innate mechanism that cleans debris out of cells (including mitochondria that have been weaned through mitophagy), clears toxins, and recycles damaged cell components. Think of autophagy as the Merry Maids of your cells. Autophagy is so important because all that cellular debris can trigger inflammatory pathways and contribute to various disease processes.

Unlike energy production, autophagy is not occurring 24/7. It is stimulated by stress and nutrient deprivation. Both intermittent fasting and exercise increase autophagy and encourage peak mitochondrial performance. We will discuss these two autophagy stimulators in practice 3 and practice 6, respectively.

As a critical component to maximizing the efficiency of your mitochondria, autophagy helps to boost energy production and combat aging, playing a key role in preventing diseases such as cancer, neurodegeneration, cardiomyopathy, diabetes, liver disease, autoimmune diseases, and infections. Autophagy and your mitochondria work hand in hand to optimize your health and expand your health span.

Stem Cells

Even though we have mitophagy and autophagy to keep our cells clean and functioning well, our cells do not last forever. When cells die or become damaged or obsolete, our stem cells replace them with new cells. Again, within the elegance of our innate intelligence there is an inborn mechanism ensuring our survival.

Each of us is born with a finite number of stem cells. They exist in every part of our body to replace cells that have died and to repair tissue damage. Stem cells are different from other cell types because they are unspecialized cells capable of renewing themselves through cell division to prevent their own depletion, sometimes even after long periods of being dormant. They can also turn into tissue or organ specific cells, such as a muscle cell, a red blood cell, or a brain cell, when prompted.

When you were a child and you got a cut or a scrape, you healed miraculously, almost overnight, because you had an abundance of stem cells. Fast forward fifty years. It can take days and even weeks to heal a cut or scrape. Your stores of stem cells have been depleted over time in response to various injuries, illnesses, infections, and lifestyle choices, resulting in a slower, diminished healing capacity. As stem cells age, their functional ability also deteriorates resulting in impaired differentiation and self-renewal. Eventually your body can no longer keep up with the demands placed on it by the environment, both internal and external, and the stressors induced by negative diet and lifestyle choices.

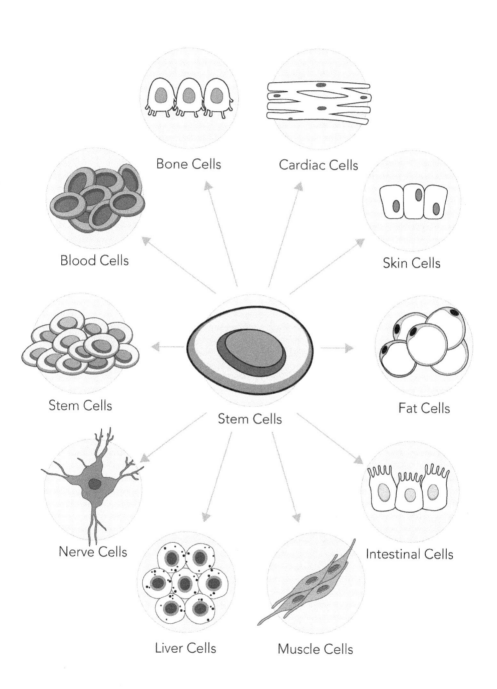

Bone Cells

Cardiac Cells

Blood Cells

Skin Cells

Stem Cells

Stem Cells

Fat Cells

Nerve Cells

Intestinal Cells

Liver Cells

Muscle Cells

Dis-ease and Stress

During my years in practice, I have come to realize that people have a major misconception about how disease happens. Commonly, people think they are healthy until the day they get a diagnosis, and then they have a disease.

This is far from the truth. We are enhancing or damaging our current state of health on a daily basis with the diet and lifestyle choices that we make. We are on a continuum, not an either/or as we have the capacity to move toward disease or toward health. We are not a stagnant environment.

As I mentioned previously, stress is at the root of disease. There are infinite sources of stress. Your brain and nervous system coordinate your body's built-in response mechanisms to combat stressors and insure your survival. These mechanisms are good. They are normal. We need them!

Inflammation and our immune response are literally life savers. They are our first line of defense. They work to prevent pathogens, like bacteria and viruses, from getting past our protective barriers, such as our skin, gut lining, and lungs. These responses work to isolate and neutralize stressors to protect the body from a systemic exposure.

Not all stress has a negative effect. Studies have shown that short-term stress and its spike of cortisol, the stress hormone, boosts the immune system. When stress forces us to adapt, increases the strength of our adaptation mechanisms, and warns us that we are not coping well and that a lifestyle change is warranted, stress then helps us maintain optimal health.

Stress, whether or not it is chemical, physical or emotional, triggers a protective response in your body. The stress can be real or perceived so there does not need to be an immediate threat, like coming face-to-face with a grizzly bear or eating a poisonous wild mushroom. You can conjure the same response by worrying about your child who has missed their curfew. Remember, your thoughts can play a profound role in the physical state of your body.

So while stress can help us, research shows that almost every system in the body can be influenced by chronic unhealthy stress. When chronic stress goes unreleased, it suppresses the body's immune system and ultimately manifests as illness. Stress can cause an asthmatic attack due to the release of histamine; it can increase the risk for type 2 diabetes by altering insulin needs; it can also increase the acid concentration in the stomach, which can lead to peptic ulcers, stress ulcers, or ulcerative colitis; and chronic stress can lead to plaque buildup in the arteries (atherosclerosis).

The health of your spine and nervous system are a key factor in determining your body's resiliency when it comes to dealing with stress. Any interference within that communication network compromises the body's ability to respond appropriately to a stressor. That interference can also be a draw on your precious and limited stem cell supply.

Stress is everywhere; no one is immune. We need to focus on reducing our exposure and elevating our coping mechanisms so we can make a course correction with our health. We will delve into stress in greater detail in practice 4. You don't have to *stress* about it now!

Change Trajectory

You can change the direction your health is headed. You have the power to take action. This book gives you the tools to build a solid foundation. I hope you take advantage of the opportunity that you have in your hand.

Research has confirmed time and time again that positive diet and lifestyle changes have a more profound and lasting effect on reversing chronic degenerative diseases and fostering health than any drug or surgery. That being said, it is far easier to prevent disease and preserve your natural resources than it is to reverse a disease process.

But it is never too late. Until it is. Sometimes, if you wait too long to make a change, it is just too late. Your body may have degenerated past the point of no return, and you may no longer have the mitochondrial performance or available stem cells to promote the degree of healing required by your circumstances. Even so, you can still experience positive benefits from making some choice diet and lifestyle changes, like dropping a few pounds and increasing your activity level and mental cognition. You can slow the degenerative process and preserve your existing level of function. But you may never normalize your diabetes or reverse your peripheral neuropathy symptoms, for example.

It was both frustrating and heartbreaking when I would have a patient come into my clinic wanting immediate relief from peripheral neuropathy foot pain. Most often the patient had a complex starting point. They were diabetic; forty pounds or more overweight; on a laundry list of medications, maybe a couple of supplements from Walmart or Costco; dealing with heart disease, not very active (because of their foot pain and resulting poor balance they would say), on a poor diet, experiencing sleep apnea, and the list goes on and on. They were hoping for a miracle and immediate pain relief because they were in crisis and at their wits end.

The reality of the situation is that their disease had been years and years and years in the making. A lifetime of choices that have been accumulating and causing a downward spiral on the disease continuum. Please work on changing your trajectory before it is too late.

You can change paths even if you live with a disease, such as diabetes. Diabetes is not your destiny unless you make it your destiny. You are not a victim; you are responsible, and you have the power to create a different outcome.

Diabetes, like most chronic degenerative disease processes, is completely manageable with diet and exercise. Yet rarely does someone heed the early warning signs and make the necessary diet and lifestyle changes. By the time that someone is labeled prediabetic they have already lost up to 50 percent of their pancreatic beta-cell function. When diagnosed as diabetic, that beta-cell compromise increases up to 80 percent. And to think this is preventable with diet and lifestyle management.

All too often the warning signs and trend alerts that your body is giving you are considered within normal limits. Treatment for diabetes is not started until you fall outside of the norm and qualify for drug therapy. But normal is not optimal and disease can be delayed and even prevented if we focus on optimal function.

Alzheimer's disease is now being called Type III Diabetes. This is again a big wake up call. It is diabetes of the brain and is both preventable and delayable. But you need to take action now, before your body has compensated and degenerated past the point of no return. Before you have damaged your mitochondria to the point of decay. Before you have exhausted your stem cells. We are remarkable, but not infallible.

Give the Body What It Needs

The body comes equipped with all of these ingenious built-in mechanisms to achieve and maintain health. We just need to make sure that we are giving the body what it needs and avoiding things that are toxic or damaging. We need to limit our exposure to those things that inhibit mitochondrial performance and prohibit autophagy. We need to protect our brain and nervous system. Sounds easy enough, but this is actually where much of the confusion and conflicting information happens.

There has been an onslaught of new technologies, supplements, and diets claiming to protect and help mitochondria to thrive, and rightly so. The focus on mitochondrial performance has been a significant anti-aging paradigm shift. The eight practices contained in this book do not rely on these innovations for success. While these techniques serve their purpose, they will be more effective if they are built on solid ground because there is no shortcut. Therefore, this book is focused on building a solid foundation.

There really is no shortcut for the eight practices contained in this book. A supplement does not replace the need for a diet full of fresh vegetables. A drug does not replace the need for sleep or exercise.

Nobody is perfect. No one's body is perfect. We practice, not perfect.

Food and Lifestyle

Oxygen, water, food, sleep, personal environment, and movement are key elements to supporting your brain and nervous system, even more specifically your mitochondria. These key elements will get you at least 80 percent of the way toward optimal health and well-being. For some people, this is all they need. For others, specific supplements and nutrients are necessary to enhance healing and assist the body in enhancing its adaptability to stress.

Health interventions should always be prioritized from least invasive to most invasive, with medication and surgery being the last resort. Trust your inborn, innate healing capacity. People do not understand how much control and power they have over their health and quality of life.

It is your personal responsibility to take care of your health. It is not the government's or an insurance company's, or your employer's, or even your doctor's responsibility. It is yours and yours alone.

Armed with that authority, remember that we vote every day with our dollars. Processed food and soda would not exist if we didn't buy it. Sure, it tastes good and it is convenient—it was created to be. It is the result of top-secret chemistry geared toward addiction.

Let's not continue to keep our heads in the sand. Health is a huge problem in your life, your children's lives, and our country. And as we have expanded our fast food to other nations, they have also been trending toward our sick and diseased statistics.

If you think that Big Food or Big Pharma has your best health interest in mind—you are mistaken. They can afford to pay out millions on class action suits and do so on a regular basis. And continue to thrive in business at your expense. The FDA's efforts are heavily funded by Big Pharma. In fact, according to an article published in Forbes magazine in June of 2018, the pharmaceutical industry provides 75 percent of the FDA's drug review budget.

There is a lot of financial incentive to keep this system going! So, don't kid yourself: you and only you have your best health interest at heart.

Furthermore, as parents, it is our responsibility to teach our children how to live a healthy life. We are their role models for eating, exercising, hydrating, sleeping, and keeping a clean home environment that minimizes toxic chemicals. I'm not perfect. My kids aren't perfect. You don't have to be perfect to achieve and maintain health. The key elements that support your brain, nervous system, and mitochondria have to be a priority and focus in your life. Having a glass of wine or a delicious French macaroon is not the end of the world. You are not a failure. The exception cannot be the rule, however.

The choices you make every day throughout your life have a cumulative effect on your internal environment. It is the string of choices that lead you toward health, or toward disease. Learning to balance what your body needs with a life rich in social connections and diverse experiences is an important aspect to success in any endeavor. It is especially true when you are striving to extend your health span and age gracefully. Now let's get started.

Part 2: The Eight Practices

"Self-care is giving the world the best of you,
instead of what's left of you"

—Katie Reed

Practice 1: Quench

Throughout my decades in practice, the most common question patients ask is, "What is the most important thing that I can do to improve my health?"

My answer has consistently been drink water. Sadly, most people do not like my simple answer.

Water is really the unsung hero of health and wellness. It is involved directly or indirectly with every cell and function in the body and makes up about 70 percent of our body weight. Water is vital for many reasons:

- Provides structure to our cells

- Transports nutrients and waste products

- Regulates temperature

- Acts as a lubricant and shock absorber

- Helps to deliver oxygen throughout the body

- Assists the brain to manufacture hormones and
  neurotransmitters

- Promotes healthy looking skin

- Assists mitochondria to produce energy.

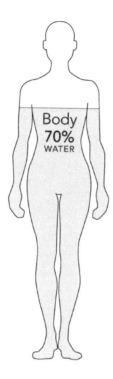

Body
70%
WATER

• Acts as a shock absorber for brain and spinal cord

• Needed by the brain to manufacture hormones and neurotransmitters

• Converts food to components needed for survival - digestion

• Forms saliva for digestion

• Allows body's cells to grow, reproduce and survive

• Regulates body temperature

• Lubricates joints

• Helps deliver oxygen all over the body

• Flushes body waste

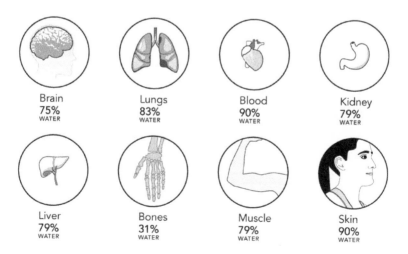

Brain
75%
WATER

Lungs
83%
WATER

Blood
90%
WATER

Kidney
79%
WATER

Liver
79%
WATER

Bones
31%
WATER

Muscle
79%
WATER

Skin
90%
WATER

Mastering the Health Continuum   39

Without water, mitochondrial performance is compromised, and aging accelerates. The water molecule touches every aspect of your health and vitality. We can only survive for a few days without water, making it the most important nutrient to influence health.

This is not new information. In fact, you are probably thinking you already know that you should be drinking water or more water.

But the fact is that you still aren't drinking enough water or drinking water appropriately for maximum hydration benefit. It is estimated that about 75 percent of Americans are chronically dehydrated. We just don't drink enough water. Let me say it again, we just don't drink **enough** water.

It amazes me that with all of the diets, detoxes, cleanses, and silver bullet drugs and supplements available on the market today, very few health innovators are promoting the foundational and profound effects that proper hydration can have on health and disease prevention. Sure, "drink water" is part of the message, but there are no inspiring insights to motivate a change in our hydration hygiene, yet water is vital to life. We haven't been set up to be successful.

Euhydration

As part of the sophistication of our innate intelligence, we have a built-in regulatory system that keeps our body water balance in check. The goal being euhydration, neither dehydrated nor overhydrated. Once proper baseline hydration is achieved, your intake and outflow of water are equal, setting your body up for optimal function and health.

Euhydration is accomplished through a complex interplay between the blood vessels, kidneys, hypothalamus in your brain, adrenal glands, and several hormones and enzymes. I am including a diagram to show the intricacy of this process.

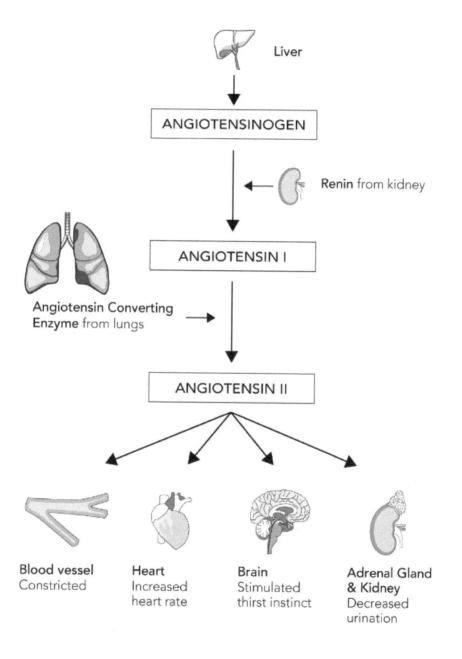

Liver

ANGIOTENSINOGEN

Renin from kidney

ANGIOTENSIN I

Angiotensin Converting
Enzyme from lungs

ANGIOTENSIN II

Blood vessel
Constricted

Heart
Increased
heart rate

Brain
Stimulated
thirst instinct

**Adrenal Gland
& Kidney**
Decreased
urination

The RAAS, renin-angiotensin-aldosterone system, is the signaling pathway responsible for regulating blood pressure. This system is important because when your water outflow exceeds your water intake, your blood volume drops, lowering blood pressure and stimulating an increase in plasma osmolality, resulting in reabsorption of water from cells and tissues to maintain blood pressure. Unfortunately, this causes concentrated urine and constipation.

We lose water through our organs by detoxification. Our gut, kidneys, skin, and lungs serve to rid our bodies of toxins and waste. When water is being reabsorbed to maintain blood pressure in response to dehydration, toxins and waste products linger in our bodies, creating an environment that predisposes dysfunction and disease. This accumulation of toxins puts added stress on our liver and lymph system. We can't expect the mitochondria in our cells to operate at an optimal level if they are swimming in toxic soup.

As you can see, a downward spiral occurs with dehydration. In a healthy, hydrated, and vital individual, these moments of imbalance are quickly corrected through the body's inborn healing mechanisms. The RAAS feeds back to the hypothalamus to stimulate thirst. Being thirsty may continue over a period of time until balance is regained.

Your body works to precisely balance hydration, a 1 percent loss of water is usually compensated for within twenty-four hours. The balance of hydration is so delicate that even a 1–2 percent decrease in body water can impair cognitive function.

Symptoms of dehydration can be mild or overt and include lack of focus, mood shifts, fuzzy thinking, and poor memory—not surprising when you consider that over 80 percent of the brain is water.

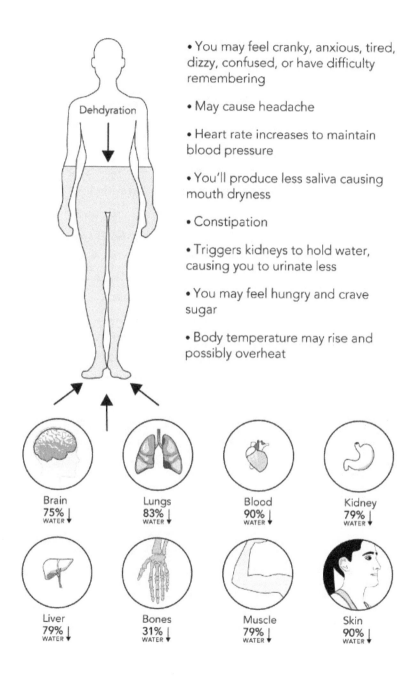

Dehdyration

- You may feel cranky, anxious, tired, dizzy, confused, or have difficulty remembering

- May cause headache

- Heart rate increases to maintain blood pressure

- You'll produce less saliva causing mouth dryness

- Constipation

- Triggers kidneys to hold water, causing you to urinate less

- You may feel hungry and crave sugar

- Body temperature may rise and possibly overheat

Brain
75% ↓
WATER ↓

Lungs
83% ↓
WATER ↓

Blood
90% ↓
WATER ↓

Kidney
79% ↓
WATER ↓

Liver
79% ↓
WATER ↓

Bones
31% ↓
WATER ↓

Muscle
79% ↓
WATER ↓

Skin
90% ↓
WATER ↓

Thirst Instinct

We have the built-in mechanism to regulate our thirst as a survival mechanism. But too often we ignore it. We have actually conditioned ourselves to ignore the thirst sensation. When we first ignore it, we are telling our brain there is no water available. That shifts us into survival mode and the brain puts the body on high alert, engaging our fight or flee response. This stimulates the body to conserve resources and hold on to what it currently has.

Survival mode slows down your metabolism causing you to have low energy, foggy thoughts, and unclear memory. It also slows your digestion and elimination, meaning you get constipated. You might even experience muscle pain or cramping. In an attempt to conserve resources, you hold on to water which may cause bloating. And now your mitochondria use sugar rather than fat to produce energy, and since survival mode stimulates your body to grow and replicate fat cells, you produce more fat and you hold on to it to ensure future survival rather than burning it for energy.

On occasion, and for brief periods of time, this disregard of the body's innate signaling mechanism has minimal long-term effects. The body compensates to use the resources it already has. But the dampening of the thirst instinct gets more complicated in our modern age.

To compound the problem of ignoring our thirst, we have become a society of sippers. We sip our coffee or tea. Unfortunately, sipping all day signals that resources, water specifically, are sparse, and then we shift to survival mode. Even though some people may even forego soda, juice, or even an artificially flavored carbonated water for an occasional glass of water, it is not enough. And no, that glass of wine, microbrew, or hard cider does not count toward your daily hydration requirements. In fact, many of society's preferred beverages actually have a diuretic effect or are heavily laden with sugar and artificial ingredients that contribute to a systemic acid shift, causing even more dehydration.

Don't get me wrong, I love a warm cup of coffee or tea, especially on dreary Northwest winter days. Enjoying a glass of wine by the fire with friends is especially gratifying. But these occasions do not replace my water; they are in addition to it.

This habit of sipping, more importantly what we are sipping, has worked to dampen our natural thirst instinct. According to a study published in 2008 in the journal of *Physiology and Behavior*, water constitutes only about 10 percent of beverage consumption. The other beverage choices supply dietary energy, meaning they contain a form of sugar. Consumption of energy-yielding beverages to relieve thirst further disrupts our homeostatic associative learning patterns. In other words, the boost of energy covers up the symptom of thirst. The sugar also stimulates a reward cascade in the brain that results in craving more sugar to replicate the boost of energy feeling.

I hope you can see where this is headed. Consuming energy-yielding beverages, those containing sugar, may help to quench your thirst; however, they do not dampen your hunger or meet your hydration threshold. This further confuses and disrupts your natural thirst instinct and your hunger instinct; thus, you may eat when you are actually thirsty. This then becomes a default behavior. So now you have learned this pattern and continue to reinforce it, and you pass it on to your children.

The hypothalamus in our brain constantly monitors our hydration, regardless of our hydration habits. A chronic state of dehydration will desensitize the brain, and we will eventually no longer get "thirsty." Through its innate survival mechanisms, the body will compensate and learns to adapt to water deprivation. It will function, but it will not function optimally. You may survive, but you will not thrive.

Aberration of these instincts may be at the root of our current obesity and cardiometabolic dysfunction epidemic as dehydration wreaks metabolic havoc. Drinking water appropriately is a simple solution to change the health trajectory of millions, if not billions, of people.

Dehydration

Unfortunately, ignoring your natural thirst instinct does not reduce your body's requirement for water and can lead to chronic dehydration. A chronic state of dehydration puts an enormous strain on the kidneys, liver, and gut, inhibiting their ability to detoxify your body.

It also disrupts the delicate electrolyte balance within the body. Electrolytes are responsible for moving electrical charges and signals through your body. This is how cells communicate with each other and how the nervous system relays information to and from your brain. When electrical signals are not transmitting properly and you are not efficiently detoxifying, it creates the perfect storm for a variety of systemic health issues. These include irregular heartbeat, allergies, weight gain, migraines, organ dysfunction, nervous system disorders, and brain fog.

The following are some symptoms that may indicate that you are chronically dehydrated:

- Dark-colored urine
- Muscle fatigue or weakness

- Infrequent urination
- Muscle or joint pain

- Constipation
- Dry eyes

- Dry or flaky skin
- Bad breath

- Headaches or migraines

Dehydration is difficult to diagnose. Symptoms can be insidious. One thing is for certain, you cannot use "thirst" as your metric for determining whether you are dehydrated or not. You have most likely lost your thirst instinct.

If you are forgetting to drink water or don't like to drink water, you are dehydrated. If you feel nauseous or sick after drinking water, this is a chronic dehydration problem that should be addressed immediately.

You may be chronically dehydrated even if you are drinking water on a frequent basis. It just might not be enough water to re-establish the proper balance required for optimal function.

Various factors can cause one to need more water. Some examples include:

- Irritable bowel syndrome

- Crohn's disease

- Diabetes

- People who live in warmer climates or high altitudes

- Pregnant women

- Breastfeeding moms

- Athletes

- Elderly people

The elderly at large suffer from chronic dehydration and a dampened thirst instinct. It is vitally important for them to be supported in proper hydration to maintain quality of life. This population in particular has the burden of a poor diet, deteriorating organ function, accumulated toxic load, and multiple prescription medications.

Various medications increase your body's water need. These medications typically increase urine output and can have side effects of vomiting and diarrhea.

- Diuretics

- Laxatives

- Chemotherapy

- Antihistamines

- Blood pressure medication

Other common medications can indirectly influence your hydration requirements. Here are a few examples of medications that directly disrupt the electrolyte balance in your body elevating your water intake needs:

- Corticosteroids   - Antifungal medication

- Birth control pills

Quality Matters

Not all water is created equal. The molecular structure is the same; however, drinking water contains more than just the water molecule. Depending on the source of your water, it can also contain heavy metals and other contaminants. All water intake increases hydration, but we don't want to create a heavier toxic burden for our bodies to try to detox.

Clean water is the goal. According to the Environmental Working Group's (EWG) tap water database, most American tap water contains industrial or agricultural contaminants linked to cancer, brain and nervous system damage, developmental defects, fertility problems, or hormone disruption. Not what we are going for!

While levels of the more than 250 contaminants identified fell within federal and state safety guidelines for the most part, they exceeded what science considers safe. What is even more disturbing is that the Environmental Protection Agency has *not* added a new contaminant to the list of regulated drinking water contaminants in more than twenty years. The EWG identified more than 160 unregulated contaminants in their study.

You can enter your zip code into the tap water database and find out what contaminants were found in your tap water and at what level. You should know what you are drinking; take responsibility. Research shows that reverse osmosis systems combined with a superior carbon filter is the best filtering system for removing contaminants. That combined with a good stainless or glass water bottle that you can fill and take with you everywhere you go will keep you hydrated with pure, clean water.

I am not a fan of plastic water bottles. Research shows that only 10 percent of those bottles, at best, get recycled, leaving 90 percent to add to our ever-growing landfill issues. In addition, plastic bottles contain bisphenol-A, or BPA, an endocrine disruptor that can wreak hormonal havoc in your body and add to your toxic burden. This is a real problem when trying to create an environment in your body to optimize health.

I will dive much deeper on plastic, toxins, and contaminants in practice 7, but suffice it to say drinking clean water, and enough of it, just might be the single most powerful habit change that you can make. It can have profound effects on your health and health span.

Optimize Your Hydration

If you find you have not been thirsty, or that you don't enjoy the taste of water, your thirst instinct has most likely gone dormant. It is simple, but not necessarily easy, to revive your natural thirst instinct. This is the most important action you can take to revitalize your body and optimize your health.

I have tried many approaches to supporting my hydration hygiene. Honestly, I achieved only marginal success from my strategies. It felt as though I had to constantly force myself to drink water, and the only way I could consume my daily quota was by basically sipping it all day. At the time I did not even consider that my natural thirst instinct had been compromised and that my approach to hydration was continuing to dampen it.

Needless to say, I was frustrated. Like many of you, I thought that I was doing the right thing. And, in fact, I was just in the wrong way.

At the peak of my discouragement, one of my business partners introduced me to Alex Charfen—not personally, although I look forward to the day, but rather to his natural thirst challenge. My life was changed.

His strategy to re-engage your thirst instinct is a systematic approach to hydration that brings you into a mode of thriving and resets your taste sensors on your tongue and in your brain, helping you to reduce your sugar cravings.

I would love to take credit for this; I really would. This program is that good! However, I am most interested in making sure that you have the best tools and strategies to get the best results. I want to set you up for success. Alex really deserves all of the credit here.

Alex Charfen's Natural Thirst Ten-Day Challenge

Your body has the power to tell you when it needs water to operate optimally, but only when it knows it's in an area of abundance. Reclaim your body's natural thirst instinct with three simple adjustments to your beverage consumption. This low-risk program is designed to give you the highest rewards in your hydration.

This is all it takes...

- Hyperhydrate: in the morning right after you get up and throughout the day

- Proximity to water: keep water with you all day

- If you think, drink: if you so much as look at your water, drink

ONE - HYPERHYDRATE (ALL DAY)

Right after you get up, hyperhydrate with at least 16 oz. (500 ml) of water. You may want to add a few drops of lemon juice and one or two shakes of sea salt for minerals.

Hyperhydrate to convince your body that water is abundant, and to prevent your body from transitioning to survival mode.

Alert your body that water is abundant all day by hyperhydrating with at least 16 oz. of water at least once every two hours. Every hour is optimal and will reawaken your natural thirst faster.

Morning Hyperhydration:

- Upon waking up, clean and rinse your mouth to lower harmful bacteria.

- Then drink as much as you can consume, ensuring it is 16–40 oz. (500-1,200 ml) of pure water—you may need to build up to these amounts.

- If you have a day where you become uncomfortable, it can indicate something else is going on with your health.

Continuous Hydration:

- Once an hour (or every two if you aren't ready for once an hour), drink at least 16 oz. (500 ml) at once to flush your body's systems and reaffirm you are in an area of abundance

TWO - PROXIMITY TO WATER

Have water with you always.

Drinking water throughout the day is difficult for some at first. But if you hyperhydrate in the morning, keep water within arm's reach at all times, and continuously hydrate throughout the day, you'll be surprised how quickly your natural thirst will become a permanent part of your life.

THREE - IF YOU THINK DRINK

Even if you just look at your water bottle, this is an indication for you to drink. Before long, you won't have to make a conscious decision to drink. Your body will crave the water it needs.

Your instinct to drink water has most likely been suppressed. Pay attention to the subtle reminders that your body gives you to drink. So much as looking at or thinking about water in any way means you should probably drink.

- Glanced at a lake, drink.

- Looked at a water fountain, drink.

- Do not miss a reminder.

PROTECT YOUR NATURAL THIRST

Eliminate all drinks other than water for ten days. By doing this, you will reduce your body's confusion around hydration, lower the resources necessary to absorb water, and increase your sensitivity to hydration. This adjustment also allows you to regain a neutral palate that is more receptive to food. To help reclaim your natural thirst, eliminate the following beverages:

- Soft drinks

- Alcohol

- Pasteurized juices

- Pasteurized milks

- Coffee

- Caffeinated or stimulant teas

- Flavored waters

- Carbonated drinks of any kind (including plain seltzer)

You can refer your friends, patients, or anyone you want to help with hydration to Alex's free ten-day natural thirst challenge: GetThirstyNow.com.

Do Not Fear the Healing Crisis

It is not uncommon to experience some side effects of rehydrating. In my experience day 3-4 are typically when symptoms occur for most people.

These side effects can include headache, nausea, diarrhea, muscle and joint pain...basically flu-like symptoms. KEEP DRINKING WATER.

This is a natural transition and these symptoms will not last.

- Be Prepared. Have water available at all times.

- Skip sipping.

- Commit to the change. Continue to drink at least ½ your body weight in ounces of room temperature water everyday.

$$\frac{\text{body}}{2} \div 8 = \text{glasses of water a day}$$

(8 OUNCE GLASSES)

This will become a habit in three–four weeks.
This habit could save your life!

Practice 2: Breathe

Breathe in. Breathe out. Repeat. This happens automatically without you having to think about it. The rate and depth of your breath is modulated by your brain and nervous system to meet the ever-changing needs of your body.

You will only survive for a few minutes without oxygen. It is that vital to your survival.

If you have ever suffered from an asthmatic attack or pneumonia, you understand the sheer panic associated with not being able to breathe, even if only for a brief period of time.

I contracted mycoplasma pneumonia when I was in my thirties. It was awful, certainly a brush with death! My family witnessed me deteriorating before their eyes. My inability to breathe in adequate oxygen quickly impacted my mitochondria's ability to produce the much-needed energy that I required to combat the infection and heal my tissues. I was a hot mess for three months.

Water and oxygen are required by mitochondria to process glucose and fatty acids in the production of ATP, the energy source used by the body. Carbon dioxide is one of the by-products in the production of ATP. It is a biochemical waste and is not recycled in the body. Therefore, carbon dioxide must be eliminated.

Because ATP is not stored in the body and is used up within seconds, we need a continual supply to meet the demands of our tissues, glands, and organs, especially the brain. This means we need a continual supply of new oxygen, as well as continual disposal of carbon dioxide.

Interestingly, the concentration of carbon dioxide stimulates the vagus nerve to alert the brain to trigger breathing, not oxygen levels. Vagus nerve activity is modulated by respiration. It is suppressed during inhalation and facilitated during exhalation and slow respiration cycles.

Now you know why you are told to take a deep breath when you are stressed out and anxious. That deep breath and its exhalation stimulate the parasympathetic nervous system to signal your body to calm down and slow down.

A Delicate Balance

Too much carbon dioxide can make the blood's pH more acidic. This can have detrimental effects on every cell and organ in the body. The brain helps to monitor and keep the blood's pH at a strict 7.4. When it drops below this and becomes more acidic, the brain stimulates the diaphragm to inspire and draw in more oxygen to balance the blood while expiring the carbon dioxide. We will talk more about pH and the body's built-in buffering systems in practice 3.

When we take a breath in, oxygen enters the lungs. We then breathe out to discard gas.

Blood from the lungs travels to the left side of the heart, whereby it is pumped through the arteries to the body. Red blood cells carry oxygen in the blood and distribute it to every single cell as they travel throughout the body.

Blood without oxygen returns to the right side of the heart through the veins. This blood is pumped into the lungs so that carbon dioxide can be released and new oxygen can be absorbed.

This happens automatically all day and all night from your first breath until your last. Can you imagine what it would be like if you had to think about every breath in and every breath out? What if you had to think about every heartbeat, to make sure that blood was circulating to distribute the oxygen and escort the carbon dioxide out? That minor change in our innate intelligence and neurology would certainly end any concern about over-population of the planet!

In addition to providing our bodies with vital oxygen, our breathing also serves to optimize information processing within our brains. Our respiratory rhythm synchronizes electrical activity in the brain. This neural synchronization has significant influence on both our cognitive function and our homeostasis regulation within the body. When stress is high, logic is low as it is difficult for the brain to take in new information and process it during stressful situations. Likewise, when stress is high, our body shifts into high alert survival mode, triggering a shift in body temperature, blood pressure, digestion, blood sugar levels, and hormone levels.

This trigger comes from the limbic system in the brain, which is responsible for regulating homeostasis within the body. It is this area of the brain that flips the switch between fight or flee and rest and restore

Rate and Rhythm

Rapid, shallow breathing stimulates the brain at a higher rate, resulting in activation of the sympathetic nervous system (flight or fight). The cascading effects include turning up stress hormones like cortisol, increasing heart rate to distribute more oxygen and clear more carbon dioxide, increasing blood pressure to circulate blood faster, and increasing muscle tension, sweat production, and anxiety. The body is being prepped to fight or flee.

Alternatively, slowing your breathing induces a parasympathetic response (rest and restore). The parasympathetic nervous system induces relaxation, calm, and mental clarity.

Our over-stimulated and stressed out population has become chronic, shallow, mouth breathers. Instead of breathing deep and slow through the nose, driving the diaphragm down into the belly, we breathe more rapid and shallow into the chest through the mouth. However, we are divinely designed to breathe through our nose. Nose breathing not only filters contaminants and warms the air to body temperature before entering the lungs, it also increases the production of nitric oxide, a potent blood vessel dilator. Nitric Oxide also opens up your airways allowing you to take more air deeper into your lungs.

Fast, shallow breathing only brings air into the upper part of the lungs where very little oxygen and carbon dioxide exchange occurs. This communicates a stress response to the brain. It stimulates the sympathetic nervous system to cause a whole-body stress response as described above. It is a vicious cycle. Moreover, shallow breathing becomes a learned habit.

Chronic shallow breathing limits the lungs performance and thus predisposes us to anatomical and physiological changes associated with the aging lung. The progressive loss of pulmonary elasticity and stiffening of the chest wall reduce the efficiency of air exchange, limiting the availability of oxygen to all of the cells in the body and also to the mitochondria. Thus, accelerating aging. Since our lungs mature by the age of twenty–twenty-five years old, our lung capacity in our later years is largely determined by peak lung function achieved during adulthood. So it is important to break the habit of chronic shallow breathing.

Chiropractic care can help to promote and maintain optimal function of the ribs and spine that surround and protect the lungs. This can help to improve poor posture, a leading contributor to shallow breathing, and promote deep, belly breathing with ease.

Air Quality Matters

The depth and rate of your breathing determines your lung capacity health and influences your stress response throughout your body. As mentioned before, there are an infinite number of stressors. Your body responds in three ways: inflammation, oxidative stress, and immune dysregulation. All three of these responses can have negative repercussions for the mitochondria in your cells and their efforts to provide you with ample energy, especially when stress is chronic or sustained. We will talk more about these three responses in practice 4.

As we breathe in approximately ten thousand liters of air each day, our lungs are directly exposed to an enormous burden of microbes and foreign chemicals that illicit a stress response.

Various lung toxins, such as nitrous oxide, tobacco smoke, ozone and air pollutants produce large amounts of ROS within the body. Remember that an imbalance between ROS and available antioxidants leads to oxidative stress. The ROS can cause direct damage to proteins, DNA, and the cell wall. Increased ROS also stimulates an influx of inflammatory cells.

Inflammatory cells release enzymes that can destroy RNA, DNA, and cell membranes. The resulting death of tissue amplifies the release of enzymes and stimulates a vicious cycle of degeneration. This breakdown in lung architecture is seen in emphysema and pulmonary fibrosis.

Both acute and chronic exposure to air pollution, especially pollution that contains particulate matter, is associated with increased risk of death from cardiovascular diseases including ischemic heart disease, heart failure, and ischemic/thrombotic stroke. Particulate matter is an important endocrine disrupter, contributing to the development of metabolic diseases such as obesity and diabetes, which themselves are risk factors for cardiovascular disease.

Additionally, particulate matter can have a negative impact on reproductive health. Exposure to polluted air, particularly vehicle exhaust, has neurotoxic implications and is associated with impaired cognitive functions at all ages and increased risk of Alzheimer's disease and other dementias in later life.

Exposure to particulate matter alters mitochondrial performance through the generation of excess ROS leading to oxidative stress and altering their DNA. Long-term particulate matter exposure leads to an increase in fat cell size and number, including the fat that surrounds your organs. It is also associated with an elevation in inflammation of this adipose, or fat, tissue. Adipose inflammation is connected with insulin resistance.

Additionally, a large portion of lung disease is caused by environmental factors, either by direct exposure to injurious agents or as the result of failure of various defense mechanisms.

Since breathing through the nose helps to filter many contaminants before they reach the lung tissue, we can change our breathing habits to increase the possibility of avoiding the aforementioned ailments.

In 2017 the *New England Journal of Medicine* published evidence supporting that there are adverse effects of exposure to particulate matter at concentrations below current national standards. The totality of the evidence suggests that there is no "safe" level of particulate matter exposure.

It is fairly easy to make the connection between exposure to pollution and resulting lung damage. However, this same mechanism causes damage in the healthy athlete who over-trains. Excessive training produces an increase in ROS that leads to chronic inflammation and tissue injury. Effects can be magnified for athletes as they run or cycle outside along roadways.

Along with contamination, your external environment can also reduce the amount of oxygen that you have available for your mitochondria (some of these include recirculating air systems, altitude, frequent travel on airplanes, and occupational hazards).

While you can't always control the external environment, you can control the air inside of your home, which may be more toxic than the outside environment. While pollutants commonly found in indoor air can cause many harmful effects, scientists are uncertain about what concentrations or periods of exposure are necessary to produce specific health problems. Some sources, such as building materials, furnishings, and products like air fresheners can release pollutants more or less continuously. Other sources, related to activities like smoking and cleaning, can release pollutants intermittently.

Usually the most effective way to improve indoor air quality is to eliminate individual sources of pollution or to reduce their emissions. The most common sources of internal air contaminants are mold, furniture, carpeting, paint, cleaning supplies, aerosol sprays, dry cleaning, and air fresheners.

Dust mites, pollen, and pet dander are common lung irritants. In addition, many hobbies utilize elements that have toxic components, such as glue, paint, and solder. Stoves, fireplaces, and heaters can contribute to internal air pollution by upping the carbon monoxide level.

Using an air filter can help to eliminate some worry about the source of all of the air toxin contributors in your home. There are many types and sizes of air cleaners on the market, ranging from relatively inexpensive table-top models to sophisticated and expensive whole-house systems. It is important to confirm that their HEPA (high-efficiency particulate air) filters are capable of capturing particles at least 0.3 microns in size. No matter which air purifier you opt for, it might surprise you just how much your health will benefit when you clean up your indoor air quality.

Limiting exposure, using an air filtration system, and wearing proper protective gear when you are knowingly exposing yourself can reduce your exposure to harmful particulate matter. This will also help to mitigate your toxic burden and remove a few stressors along the way.

Optimize Your Inspiration

Hopefully, you can see the obvious importance of nurturing your lungs and lung health. In addition to eliminating toxic exposure, proper breathing techniques and regular aerobic activity are key elements of developing, improving, and preserving lung function.

Yoga

I especially like yoga as a method for improving lung health. Yoga incorporates breathwork and breathing techniques as a way to focus the mind and the body. And it can play an important role in boosting your lung health.

There are many different types of yoga practice. The type of practice does not influence a particular result when it comes to the positive side effects that intentional breathing can have. In addition to the benefits that your lungs and cells experience from deep, relaxed inspiration, many other positive results can be seen in physical, mental, and cognitive performance.

Physical Health:

- decrease in cardiometabolic risk factors

- increase in cardiopulmonary health and fitness

- immunological improvements

- anti-inflammatory effects

- bone density, balance, strength, and flexibility

- improvement in chronic pain conditions such as migraine, fibromyalgia, and osteoarthritis

Mental Health:

- reduce multiple physiological stress markers such as heart rate, blood pressure, cortisol levels, and inflammation

- decrease in symptoms of depression, anxiety disorders, and post-traumatic stress disorder

- enhancement in brain function and memory enhancement in attentional control

Researchers have studied the effects of yoga on heart rate variability, a good measure of how stress is impacting the body, and they concluded that the rate and depth of breathing plays a significant role in determining whether the body will be on high alert waiting to fight or flee, having a sympathetic nervous system dominance, or if it will be calm, cool, and collected under the influence of the parasympathetic nervous system. Breathing stimulates the vagus nerve both directly and indirectly. Slow, deep breathing is a function of the vagus nerve and consciously breathing engages the nerve. The indirect route involves stimulation through physiological biofeedback. When you adopt the body patterns associated with relaxation and low threat situations, like slow breathing, the vagus nerve communicates this state to the brain. The brain interprets this as a low stress or threat situation and encourages a rest and restore state top-down, again through the vagus nerve. The indirect route is responsible for more long-term tonic changes of vagal tone.

Therefore, respiratory stimulation of the vagus nerve not only produces a change in parasympathetic nervous system activity during and right after yoga, it also results in a long-term tonic shift in autonomic balance. This shift is known as vagal dominance. We will talk more about this in a practice 4 and delve into the positive benefits of vagal dominance.

Breathing Exercises

The American Lung Association recommends we practice breathing exercises for five–ten minutes per day. Two of the most common breathing exercises incorporate nasal breathing. You can perform these exercises either seated or laying on your back. The nasal breathing technique increases nitric oxide levels, offering up a boost of energy.

Pursed Lip Breathing

Simply take a deep, slow, and steady breath in through your nose and breathe out at least twice as long through your mouth with pursed lips. This method helps to keep your lungs and airway expanded for a longer duration.

It is helpful to tune into your normal breathing rhythm for several breath cycles prior to starting. You may need to slowly extend your inspiration over several breath cycles. I find it works best to focus on a four-second inspiration and an eight-second exhale.

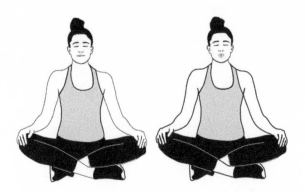

Belly Breathing

This technique works to re-engage your diaphragm. Use the same breathing method and rhythm as described above. In addition, be cognizant of your belly extending as you breathe deeply into your belly.

You may feel uncomfortable and uncoordinated initially as you likely recruited your neck and shoulders to compensate for your diaphragm with chronic shallow breathing habits, but stick with it.

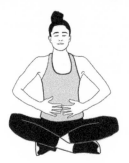

To take these exercises to the next level and create greater awareness of your breathing in general, and your diaphragmatic engagement specifically, you can try the following modifications to the above exercise. It is best to do these exercises while laying on your back.

1. Put your hands on top of one another, both palms facing toward you. Place your hands on the center of your chest just below your collar bones. Let's call this position one.

   Using the pursed lip breathing technique above, focus your breath under your hands. Complete a few breath cycles, and then move your hands a few inches lower on your chest. Complete a few more breath cycles, and move your hands a few inches lower and repeat. Continue to move your hands a few inches at a time and complete several breath cycles at each location. Finally, your hands should be right below your ribs and above your belly button. Let's call this position two. Complete a few breath cycles here, and then work your way back up to position one. Remember to focus your breath to where your hands are located.

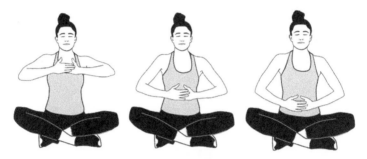

2. Resume position one. Breathe in through your nose and out through your mouth, concentrating on your chest elevating under your hands. Repeat this several times until it feels comfortable and flows easily.

   Now move your hands to position two. Again, breathe in through your nose and out through your mouth, focusing on your breath elevating your abdomen as your diaphragm pushes downward. Repeat for several breath cycles.

   Alternate between position one and position two, completing several breath cycles at each location. Remember to focus your breath on your hand location.

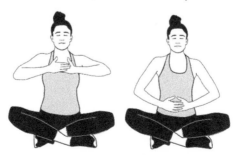

3. Resume position one. Leave your bottom hand on your chest and move your top hand to position two.

Inhale through your nose, focusing your breath on position one. Exhale slowly through your mouth.

Inhale through your nose, focusing your breath on position two. Make sure that your belly is rising underneath your hand. Exhale slowly through your mouth.

Continue to alternate your breath between position one and position two, maintain proper breathing rhythm, and keep your body relaxed.

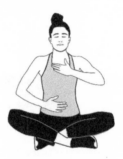

Practice Insights

- Perform breathing exercises daily.
- Limit toxic pollutant exposure.
- Invest in an air filter to help bolster the quality of air within your home.

Practice 3: Nourish

You are what you eat. Because our food has become tainted with flavorings, preservatives, pesticides, antibiotics, and hormones; and our soil is reportedly depleted of vital nutrients and minerals, we need to know where our food is coming from.

Is it being grown in rich, organic soil? Is clean water being used for irrigation? Have the seeds been altered to grow new to nature foods that are resistant to the debilitating effects of pesticides? Is it being harvested at the peak of ripeness? Or is it harvested prematurely and then enhanced with chemicals and dyes to give the illusion of the perfect specimen?

Clean food and good nutrition appear to be not only idealistic, but also seemingly unachievable. It takes hard work and diligence to maximize your nutrition and minimize your exposure to toxins. And on top of that, we are bombarded with opinions on what we should eat and what we should avoid, leaving us more confused and apathetic than before.

We live in a time when there is a new fad diet, miracle food, or supplement every month it seems. They all offer hope to the frustrated and discouraged and strive to offer a solution to our ever-growing health crisis in America. Obesity and cardiometabolic disease are reaching epidemic levels. And in spite of all of the options available to us, we continue to get fatter and sicker while our children also have to deal with a poor diet and toxic world.

There isn't a quick fix or a one size fits all answer to this growing problem. It is definitely an arduous task to sift through all of the information and science to determine what is right for you. Not only is there an abundance of information, much of it is conflicting. Unfortunately, people often rely on celebrity endorsements in their decision making, omitting their own bio-individuality: their personal and family medical history, current lab findings, current medications and supplements, and current level of health or disease.

My decades in practice has proven time and time again that if we focus on creating the optimal internal environment for your body, the answer to the question "what should I eat" will become crystal clear. Everyone's body is different. Supporting your uniqueness is the key to success in optimizing your health and expanding your health span.

What Are We Feeding?

This question may take you by surprise. There are many reasons that people eat food: to celebrate and reward themselves, to "cure" stress, to comfort them, or to feel in control. I find it odd and profound that we strive to feed our souls, but not our cells.

Emotional eating has a negative connotation. But in reality, we are all emotional eaters. Everything you put in your mouth triggers a cascade of events in your brain and body. Sugar produces a positive, feel-good response. A glass of wine serves as a de-stressor, especially at the end of a tough day.

No one wants to feel deprived, and as a result, we are unconsciously reinforcing a negative pattern of self-medicating with food. It goes something like this: drag yourself out of bed in the morning and have a cup of coffee to get you going, skip breakfast because you are not really a breakfast person, supplement your energy with more coffee until lunch, eat a big lunch because now you are "starving," grab a pick-me-up of sugar (soda, candy, latte) in the midafternoon, eat a high carbohydrate supper since you are too bushed to cook, and finish off the evening with a few glasses of wine or other adult beverage, and then you have trouble sleeping only to wake up tired and repeat the cycle.

Now that particular cycle of self-medicating behavior may not be exactly the same for everyone, but you do get the gist of it. Feeding your emotions may take on the form of late-night eating, binge eating, not eating enough, or even purging. All of these patterns are just that—patterns. Habits that you have developed over time that are now ingrained within your nervous system.

To change those patterns, we need a paradigm shift! Let's focus on feeding your cells, more specifically your mitochondria. Remember, it is the health and performance of your mitochondria that determines the rate at which you age and predisposes you to chronic degenerative and autoimmune diseases. Those mitochondria also determine your energy level.

Ultimately, your mitochondria need water, oxygen, and glucose to make energy. Seems simple enough; however, there are thousands and thousands of chemical processes that occur along the way to get those vital components into the mitochondria and available for use in producing energy.

We can make it easy on our bodies and mitochondria, but we tend to make it hard. One of the primary reasons that our mitochondria deteriorate is the over-consumption of poor quality foods and the under-consumption of nutrient dense, healthy ones. It takes more energy and resources to extract usable components from processed food and artificially engineered beverages. It takes more energy to process pesticides, hormones, and other toxins commonly associated with commercially produced food. This excess energy expenditure and exposure to toxins also produces an increase in ROS and inflammation. It's no wonder that we are sick and tired!

When it comes to feeding our cells, food is preferred over supplements. Whole foods provide a more bioavailable source of essential nutrients in a combination that nature intended. If you build a solid foundation of eating habits, you will optimize your cell function. Consequently, your metabolism will sort itself out in the process. Adaptogens and supplements can be used later to help fine tune your mitochondrial performance. However, many people achieve ideal results with diet and lifestyle alone, incorporating the eight practices within this book.

There are no medications specifically designed for mitochondria. Diet and lifestyle are by far the most effective way to bio-hack your cellular health. In order to give them what they crave, we need to first understand what an alkaline-rich environment is.

pH

A diet full of alkaline-rich foods is as basic (no pun intended) as you can get. Regardless of how hard you tried to convince your mother or grandmother otherwise, there are no valid reasons, disease processes, or conditions that contradict the consumption of vegetables. Focusing on creating an alkaline-rich diet will optimize your body function, especially your mighty mitochondria.

We all should have a basic understanding of pH from high school chemistry. It is the measure of hydrogen ion concentration that determines whether an aqueous solution will be acid or alkaline, hence the power of hydrogen. The pH scale typically runs from 0–14, with 7 being considered as neutral. A pH below 7 is acidic and above 7 is alkaline.

Our bodily fluids vary in pH depending on where they are located. Gastric acid in our stomach maintains a pH of 1.5–3.5 to effectively break down the food that we eat and kill the many pathogens that we ingest. Blood maintains a strict 7.4 pH. Our saliva and urine allow for a broader pH fluctuation and are more influenced by the foods we eat and the beverages we drink.

The biochemical activities in our bodies are highly sensitive to the concentration of hydrogen ions. Therefore, even the slightest alteration in extracellular pH can have widespread and detrimental effects on optimal cellular function. And remember, the health of your cells and mitochondria determines the health of you and the rate of your aging.

There are two main influencing factors at work on a daily basis that can disrupt the pH within your body. These are the acid by-products of normal metabolism and the acid or alkaline-producing effects of the foods you eat and the liquids you drink. If your body is in a state of slight acidosis, you may have a greater risk of developing osteoporosis, weak muscles, heart disease, diabetes, kidney disease, and a host of other health problems. Acid environments are favored by many parasites, fungi, Candida, viruses, and cancer. This is not the platform on which to produce health and optimal function.

Fortunately, we are equipped with innate mechanisms to maintain the proper pH levels in all of our tissues and organ systems. We have three main pH regulatory mechanisms in our bodies and all three need to work in concert to maintain our delicate and optimal balance.

Physiologic Buffers:

These are your rapid response chemicals, like bicarbonate, designed to be a quick fix to minor pH changes in the extracellular environment. There is not an endless reservoir of these chemicals, requiring constant replenishment.

Respiratory Acid-Base Control:

The lungs play a key role in helping to correct longer-term pH disruptions. They can efficiently eliminate carbon dioxide, a volatile acid and by-product of cellular respiration.

Renal Acid-Base Control:

The kidneys are vital to excreting excess hydrogen ions if pH is too low and generate more hydrogen ions if pH is too high. Optimal kidney function plays a big role here.

Our bodies have a pre-programmed hierarchy of importance in this regard and will diligently work to maintain homeostasis. Maintaining pH is key to survival.

In essence, maintaining life does not necessarily equate to an optimal quality of life. The complex and continual process of maintaining pH balance within our body draws upon immediately available and stored alkalizing nutrients, such as calcium, magnesium, and potassium. The depletion of these vital nutrients compromises cellular vitality, as well as bone and organ health and immunity.

If we do not have an ample amount of alkalizing minerals readily available in the body, through its innate buffering systems, it will leach those minerals out of the bone and muscle to restore and maintain its ideal blood pH. Other implications of depleting these mineral stores include sarcopenia, anxiety, aches and pains, and sleep disturbances. While a diet that is predominantly alkaline rich does not directly make your blood more alkaline (remember your body will keep blood pH steady), it does provide the essential components required by the buffering systems so your bone integrity and other physiologic mechanisms can be maintained.

Before the onset of industrialized food, our potassium to sodium ratio was 10:1. Now it is 1:3 because of the consumption of processed food, according to a review published in the *Journal of Environmental and Public Health* in 2012. Most of the research surrounding the impact of this relationship has been related to its effect on hypertension, but rest assured the effects are realized throughout every system of your body.

There is mounting evidence that pH can have dramatic effects on cell physiology. Of great importance is the impact it has on the mitochondria. Remember, the mitochondria are responsible for generating all of the body's energy needs by using oxygen and water to convert glucose and fatty acids into ATP. One of the by-products of ATP generation is ROS.

As mentioned previously, ROS can wreak havoc throughout the body through oxidative stress, apoptosis (programmed cell death), and lipid and DNA damage. ROS production has been shown to contribute to an acidic intracellular environment. The accumulation of these effects can further alter the efficiency of mitochondrial energy production, thus, increasing the production of ROS. It is a vicious cycle. All of which contribute to disease and accelerated aging.

While pH is not the only factor that determines the rate of ROS production, it is an important one. Research has shown that by increasing the extracellular pH, the intracellular pH consequently increases. An alkaline environment helps to stabilize the chemical reactions and membrane permeability that occur during cellular respiration and the electron transport chain, resulting in a substantial decrease of ROS release.

Hopefully you are realizing the importance of creating an alkaline environment to optimize cellular function and physiology. Many key factors negatively affect the pH levels in your body and your body's ability to regulate pH:

Stress

We will dive into the importance of stress mitigation in practice 4. For now, it is important to make the connection between stress and ROS. Stress, whether or not it is physical, chemical, emotional, financial, perceived or imagined induces an elevation in cortisol and an increase in ROS production through heightened demands made on the mitochondria.

Ultimately, stress can have a negative, acidic impact on the cellular environment if gone unchecked. Especially when there is not an abundance of alkalizing minerals to neutralize the pH.

Sleep Deprivation

Again, we will take a more in-depth look at the impact and importance of sleep in practice 5. Suffice it to say that sleep is when the body heals and regenerates. Lack of sleep has been identified as a primary stressor and cortisol disruptor.

Smoking

You would be hard pressed to find any positive implications of smoking. Of the numerous downsides associated with smoking, increased oxidative stress is one of them.

Cigarettes contain toxic heavy metals, including cadmium, arsenic, and lead. Because heavy metals are non-degradable, they persist in the environment. They have received a great deal of attention owing to their potential health and environmental risks. Although the toxic effects of metals can vary, it is well documented that they can cause interruptions of intracellular homeostasis including damage to lipids, proteins, enzymes, and DNA via the production of free radicals, including ROS.

Sugar

Sugar is a highly addictive drug that is subsidized by the federal government. It has been implicated in a plethora of disease processes ranging from cardiometabolic disorders to obesity. The bottom line is that it creates an acidic environment which disrupts the balance of essential minerals, increasing cortisol levels and contributing to the vicious cycle and downward spiral of aging.

We consume too much, way too much! Americans, on average, devour in excess of 150 pounds of sugar per year per capita. While soda is the most commonly consumed form of sugar by volume, sugar in all forms is the most common food additive. And while we often seek out sugar, sometimes we don't even know we are consuming it. Food scientists are ingenious at hiding sugar as there are more than sixty names for sugar on ingredient labels.

Even more disheartening, people who consume sugar tend to consume less water, vegetables, and fruit. This makes achieving health an uphill battle. Stay tuned and you will see how important "alive" food is in providing your body with the essential nutrients to keep you running on the alkaline end of the pH spectrum.

More factors inhibit proper pH balance than enhance it. The good news is that supporting an alkaline pH becomes simple. Drink water and eat lots of fresh vegetables and some fruit.

Hydration

We have already discussed the importance of hydration for your overall health and mitochondrial health (see practice 1 for a refresher).

You have been given a proven process to develop optimal hydration and establish a habit of hydration. Drink Water.

Food

Published data shows the effects of acidic and alkaline food on health. In 1995 the Potential Renal Acid Load (PRAL) of foods was published in the *Journal of American Dietetic Association*. This rating of food makes evident the correlation between our modern, industrialized, and highly addictive consumerist diet and the state of our current health affairs. It is not good. It is downright poor.

I am including a diagram so you can make a quick evaluation of your current diet. More in depth information can be found on my website at www.drnancymiggins.com. Our pre-agricultural ancestors ate a diet that was 87 percent alkaline producing food that yielded high levels of bicarbonate. The current American diet has displaced these high-bicarbonate-yielding plant foods with cereal grains and energy-dense, nutrient-poor foods—neither are alkaline producing.

Interestingly, some fruits and vegetables that we consider to be acidic, like lemons and tomatoes, actually have an alkalizing effect within the body rather than an acidic one. For this reason, please review the list closely when opting for or omitting certain foods.

Spinach
Cucumber
Kale
Avocado
Broccoli
Celery
Bell peppers
Carrots
Lemon
Artichoke
Asparagus
Radish
Onion
Zucchini
Olive oil
Papaya
Fig
Blueberries   Meat
Strawberry   Grains
Kiwi   Dairy
Orange   Sugar
Apple
Banana   ACID
Pineapple

ALKALINE

Given that an acidic environment promotes disease and dysfunction and an alkaline environment enhances the efficiency of cellular function, we just need to eat more alkalizing food and drink more alkalizing beverages.

As you can see, providing your body with the key dietary components that it needs to operate efficiently is of vital importance. pH imbalances may take years to manifest symptoms that reach clinical significance. Take action now to reverse the damage before it is too late. It is easier to prevent disease than it is to reverse it.

Optimize Your pH

Stop smoking. Period.

Measure your urinary and salivary pH to identify where you are starting from. It is eye-opening to see how your food and beverage choices impact your pH. Often times you will see your pH change before you feel differently or experience a change in symptoms. Part three will explain how to measure this.

Drink the recommended amount of water daily. Remember to avoid sipping! Review practice 1 if necessary.

Start the day with warm lemon water. It will help to prime your liver and stimulate the release of toxins that have accumulated over night. I have included my favorite recipe. (Caution: the sourness of the apple cider vinegar may take some getting used to. Start with half teaspoon if you are struggling and increase the amount to one teaspoon after a few days. Consistency is the key.)

Lemon Water
1 cup hot water
¼ lemon, squeezed
1 t raw apple cider vinegar
1-2 dashes of cayenne pepper

While enjoying your lemon water, prepare an alkalizing green drink. I drink this recipe for breakfast every day. This recipe is easy to double or triple, and the green drink will keep for up to two days in the refrigerator.

Alkalizing Green Drink

In a Vitamix, or other high-speed blender, combine:

3 cup power greens (combination of kale, spinach, and chard)

1 cup 100% coconut water

½ lemon, squeezed and discard rind

1 stalk celery

½ green apple

½ banana

½" turmeric, peeled

½" ginger, peeled

Blend

It is important to include foods that are organic and high in phytonutrients, antioxidants, and minerals. I am not going to tell you what to eat specifically. You are unique in this regard, and figuring it out yourself will heighten your consciousness and intuition when it comes to feeding your cells. I will make general recommendations and give examples, but it is ultimately up to you to do the work.

Eat 80 percent alive alkaline-rich food. It is important to eat a wide variety of vegetables and fruit. I have had patients who did not "like" vegetables try to eat only spinach or broccoli. That is a good place to start, but you will not realize your health goals or health potential without eating plenty of diverse vegetables. Be adventurous, try new foods. Experience the rainbow!

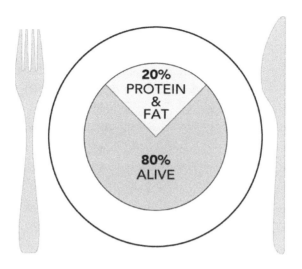

Strive to eat ten servings of vegetables and two servings of fruit daily. You don't have to specifically measure your servings, Mother Nature has done the heavy lifting for you. In general, one piece of fruit, like an apple or banana, is a serving. Consider one half cup the serving size for berries, grapes, and melon. Same for vegetables: one normal sized carrot or a stalk of celery is a serving. You need about one cup of raw, green leafy vegetables or one half cup steamed to make one serving. Consume at least 50 percent of your produce in its raw form.

If you are concerned about sugar, which most of us should be, you can use the glycemic index as a guide in conjunction with PRAL. The glycemic index assigns a value to food based on how quickly it increases blood glucose. Foods low on the glycemic index scale tend to release glucose slowly and steadily. Foods high on the glycemic index release glucose rapidly. I recommend staying on the middle to lower end of the scale primarily. The important thing to remember is to eat lots of vegetables. The green drink meets three servings of vegetables and one serving of fruit of the recommended daily consumption, and it is all raw.

As your pH increases and becomes more alkaline, your cravings for sugar and carbs will decrease; your energy will stabilize; and you will have abundantly more energy than you did while eating processed food and loads of sugar.

Protein and healthy fat should comprise 20 percent of your food daily. Protein is essential for your body. While vegetables do contain some protein, legumes, nuts, seeds, eggs, fish, and other meat are also great sources. It is extremely important to consume only clean, organic grass-fed meat. You do not need to continue to expose your body to the pesticides, hormones, and toxins that accumulate within the fat of the meat. Always avoid farm-raised fish, including salmon, tilapia, and shrimp. In practice 7 we discuss toxic burden and its effect on you and your mitochondria. Again, look to the PRAL for choices that will support an alkaline environment in your body. Fat is especially important for your brain, nerves, and cell membranes. Some healthy examples include extra virgin olive oil, avocado, and coconut.

I do recommend avoiding dairy and processed grains, including the gluten-free variety. Lots of people have an issue with this and struggle with eliminating these items from their diet. Don't shoot the messenger. I can tell you that as you increase your alkalinity, it will be easier for you to let go of these things. And if you can't or absolutely don't want to, there is no shame in that. As long as you are eating ten servings of vegetables every day and being properly hydrated, you will see a world of difference for your health.

Try to confine your eating to an eight- to ten-hour period, allowing for an extended fast overnight. It is highly beneficial to complete your food intake at least three hours prior to going to bed. Remember, autophagy is stimulated by calorie restriction. Strong research supports the benefits of restricted eating and intermittent fasting on the health and performance of your mitochondria.

- Feed your cells.
- Eat ten servings of vegetables every day and two servings of fruit.
- Focus on increasing your pH.
- Eat organic to avoid toxins. The EWG publishes a Dirty Dozen and Clean Fifteen list each year to identify which fruits and vegetables should absolutely be eaten in the organic form and those that are clean enough to eat from a standard commercially produced source.

Practice 4: Zen

Stress

Relaxation seems more of an idea or concept rather than an actual practice these days. Practicing the art of relaxation is a luxury that most of us claim to have no time for.

The reality is that we all have twenty-four hours in a day and seven days in a week. While we all have an abundance of stressors that we fall victim to, it is essential to gain control and effectively reduce and manage these stressors. Your life depends on it!

Considered the "father of stress," Hans Selye defined stress in 1936 as a state characterized by a uniform response pattern, regardless of the particular stressor, that could lead to long-term pathologic changes. He described stress as "the non-specific response of the body to any demand for change." Stress, whether or not it is physical, chemical, or emotional, real or perceived puts additional demands on the body and alters its function.

Our adaptability and resiliency largely determine the long-term impact that stress has on our bodies.

Many situations can cause stress, not just physical threats:

-Exposure to hot or cold temperatures

-Dehydration

-Starvation

-Bacteria, viruses, and pathogens

-Gluttony

-Perceived threats

-Fear

-Worry

-Sleep deprivation

Stress, in general, is considered to be negative, often synonymous with distress. Consciously, stress is the perception that the demands placed on you exceed your capacity and resources to respond to those demands. Distress typically brings to mind loss of a loved one, divorce, death of a pet, an emotionally toxic work environment, or getting a terrible diagnosis. But it can also be associated with situations like moving, getting married, and transitioning jobs.

Two factors primarily determine your response to stressful situations: how you perceive the situation through your internal map of reality and your general state of physical health, which is largely determined by your lifestyle choices. The consumption of tobacco and alcohol, dietary choices, and toxic burden as well as how often you exercise directly impacts your health and influences your ability to respond appropriately to stress. In addition, any physical pressure on the nervous system that interferes with the communication between your brain and body, and vice versa, can decrease your nervous system's resiliency and negatively impact your ability to respond appropriately to the stressors in your life.

Not all stress is bad. Stress can help to improve your performance. It can be helpful and good when it motivates people to accomplish more. It can make you run faster, work harder, and elevate your determination and tenacity. This good stress is what Hans Selye called eustress.

Eustress keeps us excited about life. Boredom and depression would certainly set in if you didn't garner anticipation and motivation. My favorite experiences of extreme eustress include riding the rollercoaster at New York-New York Hotel and Casino in Las Vegas, bungee jumping in Colorado, skiing double black diamond runs, and windsurfing in Maui. Milder forms of positive stress might be watching a scary movie, the first day at a new job, a first date, or first kiss. All of these examples encompass a blend of excitement, fear, and a sense of accomplishment. And they all generate an acute stress response.

OUR INTERNAL MAP OF REALITY

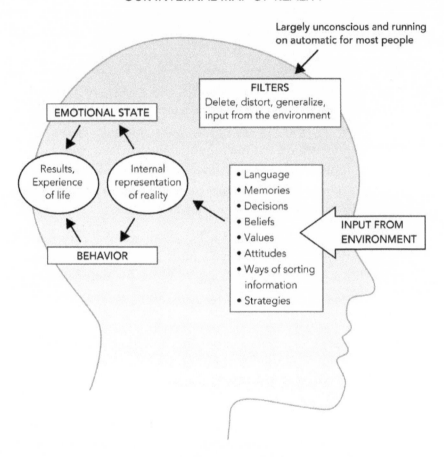

Courtesy of Centerpointe Research

Increased stress can result in increased productivity, up to a point. That threshold differs for each of us. For some, pushing up against this threshold means excitement and challenge, good stress. For many others, it conjures an undesirable state of chronic fatigue, worry, and frustration, and an inability to cope. When you reach your threshold, the signs and symptoms can be so subtle that you often ignore them. You may ignore those signals; however, you can bet that others around you are aware that you are experiencing stress overload before you are. This downward spiral is insidious.

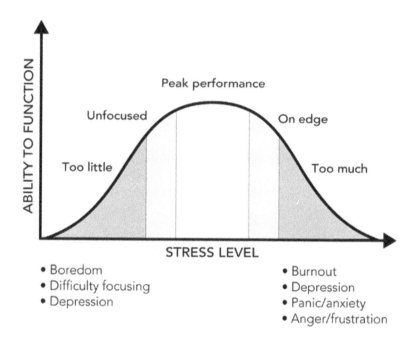

Ideally, we adapt along the way and can keep the stress response in check. Allostasis, this ability to achieve stability through change, is key to our survival. A healthy body and nervous system can have that level of resiliency. Through allostasis the autonomic nervous system, the hypothalamic–pituitary–adrenal (HPA) axis, and the cardiovascular, metabolic, and immune systems protect the body by responding to internal and external stressors.

However, most often we are not keeping stress in check. We feel that we can "handle it," persevering to meet the demands placed on us and ignoring the damage to our health and performance. But if you really hone in on your behavior and pay attention, you will inevitably see that instead of "handling it," you are employing strategies to compensate for the ever-increasing load of stress. Innate mechanisms work behind the scene compensating in an effort to maintain balance. The price of this accommodation to stress can be an allostatic overload, the wear and tear that results from chronic overactivity or underactivity of allostatic systems.

The Stress Response

In contrast to homeostatic systems, such as blood oxygen/carbon dioxide and blood pH, which must be maintained within narrow ranges, allostatic systems have much broader boundaries. Allostatic systems are flexible and enable us to respond and react to our physical states. They are constantly adjusting our physiology to account for when we are awake versus asleep, standing versus laying down, and exercising instead of sitting in front of a computer. They also work to help us cope with noise, crowds, danger, and infections. The core of the body's response to a challenge is twofold: turning on an allostatic response that initiates the appropriate adaptive pathway and shutting off this response when the threat is past.

We want flexibility within our autonomic nervous system, allostasis. A balance that allows for an appropriate stress response when warranted and an ample time spent in a calm, zen state that promotes healing. These two states cannot exist in the same moment. The nervous system is designed to fluctuate its control back and forth between the sympathetic nervous system and the parasympathetic nervous system in response to the stress in the environment, both internal and external, perceived or real. This fluctuation relies on clear and open communication via the nerves; if there is any nerve interference, a source of chronic stress, the nervous system tends to get locked into a sympathetic dominant state.

The hypothalamus is the gatekeeper. This area of the brain determines whether the sympathetic nervous system or the parasympathetic nervous system is stimulated. The vagus nerve is the primary way that the brain performs parasympathetic activities in the body. It has a vast network of connections bridging communication between the brain and vital organs.

A complex interplay between the nervous system and endocrine system incorporates three key components involved in controlling the body's innate stress response. The hypothalamus, pituitary gland, and adrenal glands are collectively called the HPA axis.

The HPA axis works in the following manner. The hypothalamus in the brain releases corticotropin-releasing factor (CRF), a hormone that binds specifically to a receptor in the pituitary gland, in response to a stressor or potential stressor.

When CRF binds to the receptors in the pituitary gland another hormone is released, adrenocorticotropic hormone (ACTH), which then binds to receptors in the adrenal glands. This results in a release of cortisol, the well-known stress hormone. The increased level of circulating cortisol in the blood ultimately feeds back to the hypothalamus, effectively turning off the release of CRF. This allows the body to return back to its normal, resting state.

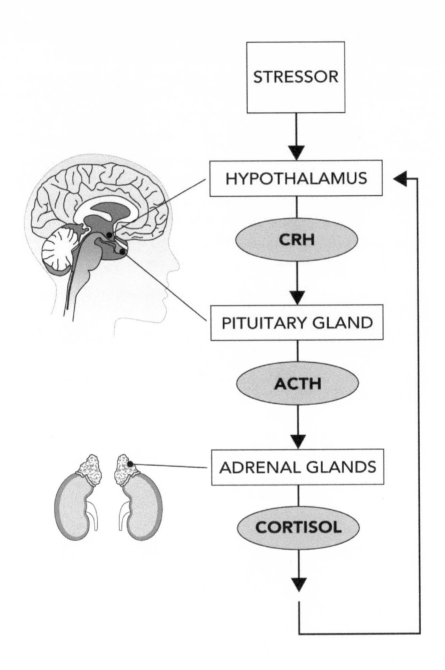

This HPA axis is responsible for the neuroendocrine adaptation component of the stress response. Three other allostatic mechanisms respond to acute stress:

1. Inflammation

Inflammation stimulates many different immune system cells. These cells release inflammatory mediators, which cause smaller blood vessels to dilate so more immune system cells can get to the injured tissue and begin the healing process. Pain, redness, and swelling are common effects of inflammatory mediators.

Infections, wounds, and any damage to tissue would not be able to heal without an inflammatory response. That being said, chronic inflammation can eventually cause several diseases and conditions including some cancers, inflammatory bowel disease, rheumatoid arthritis, and atherosclerosis.

2. Oxidative Stress

Oxidative stress occurs when we don't have enough antioxidants to neutralize the ROS being produced. This accumulation of ROS damages the mitochondria which ultimately results in an increased production of ROS. It is a vicious cycle. If left unchecked, it can result in irreversible mitochondrial decay, accelerated aging and deterioration of the body.

3. Immune Dysregulation

The immune-enhancing effects of acute stress are the result of cortisol and last for three to five days. Acute stress has the effect of signaling immune cells to be on high alert.

The immune system is divided into an innate immune system and an adaptive immune system. The innate immune system, along with various tissue barriers, is our first line of defense. It does not require previous exposure to an invader to institute its defenses. The adaptive immune system, on the other hand, is more specific and utilizes specialized methods to identify an invader's uniqueness and assign antibodies and anti-inflammatory cells to neutralize it. It also remembers the invader in case of a future attack. General immune dysregulation, commonly from persistent stimulation or compromise of a tissue barrier, leads to compensatory and exaggerated chronic inflammatory responses that result in tissue damage and autoimmunity.

Every system of the body responds to acute challenges with allostasis leading to adaptation. One response may signal the other responses to engage. Repeated exposure to stressors desensitizes the feedback response, resulting in sustained cortisol release. When your body receives an inadequate allostatic response like this, it triggers other allostatic systems to compensate with overactivity. For example, if cortisol secretion does not increase in response to stress, secretion of inflammatory cytokines, which are counter-regulated by cortisol, increases thereby increasing inflammation.

All of this is normal and desired; it is through these innate response mechanisms that our body protects us and ensures our survival—except in the case of chronic or sustained stress. When acute responses are overused or inefficiently managed, allostatic overload results. This allostatic overload can have many negative effects on the body.

A chronic state of stress creates an imbalance in our autonomic nervous system and desensitizes its innate response mechanisms. This was once coined "adrenal fatigue," but modern science has now recognized this imbalance to encompass the entire HPA axis, not just the adrenal glands.

In this state, mental functions like learning, problem solving, and reasoning are inhibited because the flight or flee response takes blood away from the brain. Remaining in this heightened stress condition for an extended period not only impairs cognitive function, it also enhances fear conditioning. Fear begets more stress. When stress is high, logic is low! Now you know where that brain fog might be coming from.

Stress, otherwise known as allostatic overload, is at the root of most of our chronic degenerative disease processes that ail so many Americans. Diabetes, heart disease, cancer, Alzheimer's disease, Parkinson's, and even arthritis, irritable bowel disease, and fibromyalgia have inflammation and oxidative stress at their core.

Chronic stress kills! It really does. Most often it is a slow subtle death, one cell at a time.

Chronic stress often triggers the eating of comfort foods that are high in fat and sugar. The impact of this allostatic load has been correlated with visceral adiposity, insulin resistance, low high-density lipoprotein levels, high blood pressure, increased triglyceride levels, reduced bone and muscle mass, decreased aerobic capacity, immune suppression, and impaired memory. All of which are associated with early onset mitochondrial dysfunction and are factors that significantly limit your health span and accelerate the rate at which you are aging.

Optimizing Your Zen

Now is the time to break the cycle and reclaim your health and healing potential.

High vagal activity, as measured by greater heart rate variability, independently predicts reduced risk of chronic degenerative disease processes and a better prognosis for those people who have already been diagnosed with a chronic degenerative disease. Heart rate variability is a measurement which indicates the variation of your heartbeats within a specific timeframe. Low heart rate variability occurs when the intervals between your heart beats is constant. If your intervals are irregular, you have a high heart rate variability.

We want high heart rate variability. This is a key metric to monitor your stress. Having a high variability means that your body is adapting and recovering from the daily stressors you are exposed to. Low variability means that you are experiencing allostatic overload and need to take action now to minimize your stressors and work to heal your body

Vagal nerve activity is also related to frontal brain activity which regulates unhealthy lifestyle behaviors. This plays a huge role when you set out to make any diet and lifestyle habit changes. When you lack vagal dominance, you tend to make poor diet and lifestyle choices. Focusing on activities that create vagal dominance and increase heart rate variability just might be the missing link in supporting you in reaching your health goals!

It is difficult to measure your actual heart rate variability without technology. For you early adopter technology geeks, see the practice insights below for a link to the Oura ring. In the meantime, you can use your resting heart rate as a gauge of stress load and recovery efficiency.

How to Measure Your Resting Heart Rate

Your resting heart rate is an important number to know and monitor. To determine your resting heart rate, measure your pulse first thing in the morning before getting out of bed. Do this several mornings in a row to get an average.

You can determine your resting heart rate by locating the pulse in your wrist and counting the beats for ten seconds, then multiplying this number by six. Ideally you want your resting heart rate to fall below sixty beats per minute.

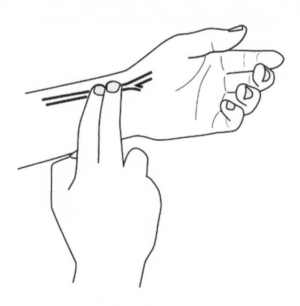

Remember that you want to increase your vagal dominance. If your resting heart rate is high, you have low vagal activity and your sympathetic nervous system is calling the shots, namely stress.

It is important to track your resting heart rate daily. If your resting heart rate is elevated even by 5 percent, you are not recovery from stress effectively. You may need more water, sleep and nutrients to support your brain and nervous system. You definitely don't need more stress!

While all eight practices are factors that can influence the vagus nerve and increase heart rate variability, this practice is most important. Stress is the root cause of all dis-sease. Remember, your brain and nervous system control and coordinate all of the activities in your body. If your brain and nervous system are not functioning at an optimal level, there is no chance whatsoever that your body can.

Achieving zen on a daily basis, just like the rest of the eight practices, is relatively simple. However, it is not easy.

Chiropractic

Chiropractic provides an answer to optimizing the communication between your brain and your body. It works to remove the interference within the nervous system by identifying where the compromise is and then correcting it. There are many chiropractic techniques available to make these corrections, including ones that are gentle and safe for infants and children.

Chiropractic care goes beyond treatment of back pain or headaches. It increases the nervous system's resiliency and promotes optimal communication and vagal dominance. Thus, it is a foundational element for anyone that experiences stress or allostatic overload, which equates to pretty much everyone.

As I stated above, you can choose from many different techniques. When working with patients that were experiencing the wrath of stress, I tended to gravitate toward low-force techniques rather than the more physical forms of manipulation. My goal being to calm everything down, not amp up a system that is already experiencing overload. Find a chiropractor that is willing to work with you to reduce the stress and pressure on your nervous system and provide you with periodic checkups to optimize your nervous system performance.

Calming the Brain

Meditation helps to unify the brain and lower the frequency of brain waves throughout the entire organ, thus, providing an ideal situation for whole-brain integration of information from our internal and external environments. Better processing of information equates to a better stress response. Meditation, even in the guided format, was difficult for me for a variety of reasons. I could not seem to effectively quiet my mind. I constantly questioned whether I was doing it properly. I frequently was interrupted. I didn't realize benefits quick enough to encourage me to continue investing the time. So I applaud those of you who have mastered meditation and are enjoying the fruits of your labor.

Interestingly enough, my experience was consistent with the feedback that I received from patients and friends. As a result, I searched for other options and started to experiment with brain wave entrainment devices. This has been a game-changer for me!

Within the first couple of weeks of use, I was sleeping better and my focus had improved. My daughter started to use the device when she studied for tests and it reduced her study time significantly, especially in the realm of memorization.

I wanted to see firsthand how this technology actually influenced the brain and neurology to calm the body and mind. Fortunately, I had the opportunity to work with an early innovator in this field, the late Rayma Ditson-Sommer, PhD. Her practice focus was twofold. She worked with elite athletes of Olympic and professional caliber, helping them to achieve "the zone" and elevate their performance. She also invested herself heavily with reactive attachment disorder children.

She held an annual summer camp for the children in her practice, and I volunteered to help at the camp; it was an eye-opening experience. These children were products of horrendous physical and mental abuse. Their innocence was lost, and the impact of the stress that they had endured (or were currently enduring) had left them struggling with behavior and learning challenges, as well as the physical manifestations of mitochondria dysfunction.

It was amazing to witness the transformation that these children experienced during those two weeks with just twenty minutes a day using the brain wave entrainment. After using the device, the kids were calm and focused and were able to process directions and express themselves clearly with words.

I also noticed changes in my own adaptability and resiliency regarding stress load. This led me to share the technology with my dear friend and mentor, Dr. Frank Sovinsky. Together, using his coaching clients as lab rats, we started measuring brain waves with an electroencephalograph (EEG). We measured brain waves before using the brain wave entrainment technology, noting left or right hemisphere dominance. Then we measured again after twenty minutes of entrainment, again noting hemisphere dominance.

It is common to favor one hemisphere over the other. Typically, right-handedness is associated with left hemisphere dominance and left-handedness is associated with right hemisphere dominance. If someone is very logical and detail-oriented, they have more left hemisphere activity. Creative types tend to have more right hemisphere activity.

Many learning challenges, such as difficulty with auditory or visual processing, can be associated with a mixed dominance. This occurs when a right-handed person is also right brain hemisphere dominant. Or a left-handed person is left brain hemisphere dominant.

Equalization, or better yet synchronization, of the brain's two hemispheres is the desired outcome with meditation. Synchronization promotes plasticity and resiliency within the brain, allowing for the appropriate fluctuation between the sympathetic and parasympathetic nervous systems in response to the stressors in our daily lives.

We confirmed that after using the technology, 100 percent of our peers tested achieved equalization of hemisphere activity. Also, it became evident that those people that used the technology daily grew to have less lateralization and quicker equalization of hemisphere activity.

Better yet, we measured their brain waves while they problem-solved, assessing hemisphere lateralization. Daily use of the brain wave entrainment technology resulted in less lateralization during the task and a more uniform engagement of the brain as a whole.

Slowing down the brain's activity is key to this synchronization process. **Brain waves** have been categorized into four frequencies, each with its own associated characteristics.

Brainwaves

Beta: Responsible for concentration, alertness, arousal, and cognition.

Higher levels are associated with fight or flight response and anxiety.

Alpha: Increases serotonin production which contributes to relaxation, calming of the mind, focus, and super-learning.

State of pre-sleep or pre-wake drowsiness.

Theta: Induces REM sleep and increased creativity.

Integrates experiences and increases openness for learning.

Increases production of catecholamines, chemicals which are vital for memory and learning.

Deep meditation.

Delta: Deep dreamless sleep and loss of body awareness.

Human Growth Hormone is released for growth and repair of the body.

Greatest influence for brain enhancement.

Each area or region of the brain generates communication signals at a specific frequency based on the predominant neurotransmitter produced in that area. In essence, brain waves are the internal communication system of the brain. Remember, when stress is high, logic is low. In a chronic stress state, the brain tends to be locked into beta wave frequency. A shift to alpha wave frequency helps to calm the mind and triggers a parasympathetic transition. Furthermore, encouraging the brain to optimize the time it spends in delta wave frequency will bolster your human growth hormone, release and foster growth, and repair your body.

Binaural Beats

Brain wave entrainment uses binaural beats. A beat pattern created by the interference pattern of separate sound waves, equal to the difference in frequency of the two sound waves. The sounds enter as separate inputs, one in each ear. The brain must reconcile the slight difference in frequency between the two tones. To do this, it creates a third tone which acts like a tuning fork, causing brain waves to synchronize. A phenomenon that scientists call entrainment.

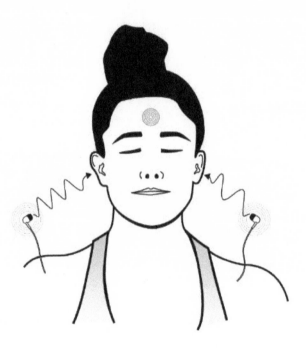

I want to clarify that entrainment is different than manipulation. Some of the binaural beat products focus on "putting" you in a particular brain wave state, which doesn't foster brain health or growth.

I have used several brain wave entrainment technologies on the market. While they each had positive elements that I appreciated, they also possessed aspects that made them difficult to use. I am a hands-down fan of Holosync in particular. The difference with this technology is that it "leads" your brain, encouraging it, rather than "pushing" you into a particular brain wave state. Bill Harris, Holosync creator and innovator in the field of brain synchronization, bolstered its effectiveness with lots of research, honing in on the most effective and efficient means to accomplish lasting results and real brain function change.

These binaural beats help guide the brain to synchronize and encourage it to reorganize at a higher-operating threshold. This threshold is largely determined by stress.

Therefore, as your brain hemispheres become more synchronized and resilient, your capacity to react and deal with stressors improves and becomes more efficient. Cortisol levels will decrease. Vagal dominance will ensue.

What I really like about Holosync is that it is subtle in every way. The binaural beats occur beneath the pleasant sound of rain and chimes. Many of my patients and friends that have used this technology say that the shift to being calm and focused is gentle and effortless. Results occur physically in your brain before you are aware that any change has occurred.

It is a proven system that can help you achieve immediate results. Using binaural beat technology in conjunction with monitoring your resting heart rate, getting frequent chiropractic checkups, and implementing the other seven practices in this book will foster an expansion of your state of zen.

Practice Insights

- Stress is at the root of disease.
- Chiropractic is effective in optimizing nervous system communication and promoting high heart rate variability.
- The Oura ring uses smart technology to collect your key personal metrics daily, including your resting heart rate and your heart rate variability. We will talk more about Oura in the next practice when we dive into sleep.
- Not all binaural beats are created equal. Seek entrainment, not manipulation.
- Always wear headphones. The binaural beats will only influence your brain if they enter each ear separately so that your brain can create the third, synchronizing tone.
- Holosync Program information can be found on my website at www.drnancymiggins.com.

Practice 5: ZZZ

Sleep, Who Needs It

Sleep is all the rage right now. And with good reason! Sleep has been an underrated enhancer of health; it is about time that it gets the spotlight. Much to the chagrin of workaholics and those who like to burn the candle at both ends, sleep hygiene is a potent determinant of our health and health span.

According to the Center for Disease Control, an estimated 84 million Americans do not get enough sleep. Our society has become tired and wired because they do not allow themselves enough time for sleep or they experience insomnia.

The American Academy of Sleep Medicine reports that insomnia occurs in up to 50 percent of adults. Insomnia does not always mean that you are bright-eyed and bushy-tailed all night while the rest of the world sleeps. It can, however, involve having trouble falling asleep, staying asleep, waking up frequently during the night, waking up too early, or waking up feeling unrefreshed. With this broad encapsulation of symptoms, it is no wonder that fatigue is one of the more common complaints communicated during clinic visits.

Sleep is not a luxury. Rather, it is a necessity. Your body cannot heal or grow without ample quality and quantity of sleep. The duration and quality of sleep affects all of the organs, tissues, and cells of the body. Mental function, digestion, hormonal balance, physical performance, and immune system function are all influenced by sleep.

The commitment to mastering sleep will bolster the overall benefits you gain from all of the other seven practices in this book.

On the other hand, sleep deprivation will sabotage your efforts and results on every level. Sleep is both a kingpin and a synergizer.

Falling asleep and staying asleep may seem like a lofty aspiration, especially since it is an extremely vulnerable act as you surrender both physically and consciously. Submission on this level is made more difficult with the onslaught of physical, chemical, and emotional stress that we are exposed to on a daily basis. I am so envious of those people that can fall asleep in seconds and get good, quality sleep just about anywhere. You know the type, or maybe it's you, that has the ability to "sleep like a baby." Oblivious to the world around them, they surrender deep into the depths of delta waves.

For more than half of my life, I lovingly referred to myself as "a non-sleeper." I have struggled my entire life with sleep. My parents tell stories of me as an infant child roaming the house at all hours of the night. Back then having your child sleep with you in bed was frowned upon. Recently, my parents told me that the doctor insisted that they "not let me win this battle." My parents' strategy was to leave the side of my crib down so I wouldn't injure myself climbing out. They figured I would eventually fall asleep when I got sufficiently tired or bored. I usually ended up at the foot of their bed curled up on a rug.

My dad is a non-sleeper as well. He worked shift work for most of his life, which really wreaked havoc on his circadian rhythm. As a young boy he was also tasked with keeping the wood stove burning throughout the night as that was the only source of heat during the frigid northern Minnesota winters. This habitual intermittent sleep interruption has been carried through this life, resulting in a deeply ingrained rhythm that wakes him during the night to this day.

Some of us are just wired this way. No pun intended! The bottom line is that sleep is essential. Lack of it can have dire consequences.

It has taken me most of my lifetime to conquer sleep. It takes discipline; however, non-sleepers can conquer their sleep. Read on and take action now. Proper sleep hygiene can help to slow down the rate at which you are aging and put your body back on the trajectory toward health.

Rhythms of Sleep

Our circadian rhythm is the predominant regulator of our sleep-wake cycle. It is present in cells throughout the body and influenced by light. When light hits the retina in your eye, it stimulates the suprachiasmatic nucleus (SCN) located in the hypothalamus of your brain. The SCN controls the timing of the sleep-wake cycle and also coordinates this with physiologic rhythms in other brain areas and tissues of the body.

Sleep is much more complex than just being asleep or being awake. There are actually four phases of sleep, the first three phases are considered non-REM sleep and the fourth phase is REM. The typical sleep cycle lasts about ninety minutes. Your goal is to average at least five sleep cycles per night or thirty-five per week if you are a healthy and well-rested individual.

While you are sleeping, your body and brain are hard at work. During sleep, you consolidate your memories, improve your learning, stimulate your creativity, and balance out your hormones and neurotransmitter, and on top of that, your body is working to repair and grow on a cellular level.

This process of growth and repair is more specifically referred to as autophagy and mitophagy. Autophagy is the process by which cellular components are cleaned up and recycled within the cell. Mitophagy is the clearance of exhausted mitochondria by autophagy.

As we discussed previously, autophagy is essential for normal cellular survival and activity. It plays a key role in aging and your health span. Disruption of sleep is connected to less optimal metabolic function and decreased mitochondrial performance. In addition, this interruption of autophagy is associated with a broad range of pathologies such as neuronal degeneration, inflammatory diseases, and cancer progression.

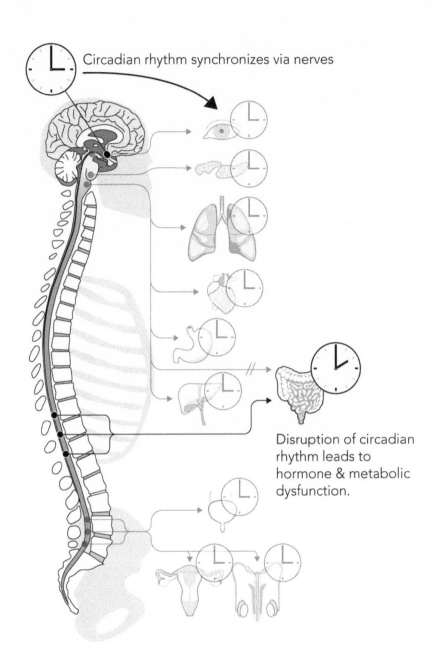

Circadian rhythm synchronizes via nerves

Disruption of circadian rhythm leads to hormone & metabolic dysfunction.

Sleep Phases

Phase 1: awake and resting

This phase only lasts a few minutes. It is the time when your brain waves, heartbeat, and breathing slow down. As your muscles relax, you might experience occasional twitching. Your brain has switched from producing the beta brain waves associated with alertness to alpha brain waves that conjure relaxation.

Phase 2: light sleep

You spend more of your repeated sleep cycles in phase two sleep than in other sleep phases. Everything continues to slow down and your body temperature drops in this phase as your brain starts to produce delta brain waves.

Phase 3: deep sleep

Healing and regeneration are stimulated in this phase. This is the period of peak human growth hormone release. Your brain is generating delta waves.

Phase 4: REM sleep

Most dreaming and memory consolidation occur during this phase. You spend more time in this phase during the early twilight hours as your brain generates theta waves.

Consequences of Sleep Deprivation

Sleep deprivation produces an allostatic overload that can have deleterious consequences. Beyond mental fatigue, not getting sufficient sleep is now considered one of the most significant lifestyle factors that influences your likelihood of developing Alzheimer's disease. While you are sleeping, autophagy is working to clean the brain of toxic debris, including the beta-amyloid protein which forms plaquing in the brains of Alzheimer's sufferers. Autophagy kicks in during sleep because you are not eating and calorie restriction is the primary trigger for autophagy. Without sufficient sleep, you fail to get that power cleanse of your cells and not just the ones located in your brain.

Moreover, according to Matthew Walker, the author of *Why We Sleep* and director of the Center for Human Sleep Science at the University of California, Berkeley, it only takes one night of insufficient sleep, getting only four–five hours, to decrease your natural killer cells (the ones that attack the cancer cells that appear in your body every day) by 70 percent. A lack of sleep is linked to cancer of the bowel, prostate, and breast. The World Health Organization has classed any form of nighttime shift work as a probable carcinogen. Mr. Walker confirms that no aspect of our biology is left unscathed by sleep deprivation.

As you can see, the effects of insufficient sleep, whether or not you get poor quality sleep or just not enough, go beyond feeling tired and fatigued the next day to damaging us on a cellular level, creating a state of chronic stress and spiraling into inflammation, oxidative stress, and immune dysregulation. We learned in the previous chapter about the toll that chronic stress takes on our health and vitality.

And so, the vicious cycle continues. There is strong evidence that insufficient sleep leads to metabolic disruption including insulin resistance and cardiovascular disease. It also promotes unhealthy food choices, eating habits, and obesity. Poor sleep can also compromise the gut microbiome, the colony of bacteria that inhabits your bowel, which can have global consequences throughout the body.

Your food choices directly impact your sleep and microbiome. This can be a difficult cycle to break. When you aren't sleeping well, you self-medicate by making poor food choices, both the foods you choose and the time you choose to eat it. These poor food choices leave you aching and craving more, making it difficult to sleep well.

Sleep Disruptors

In addition to stress and poor diet, a number of sleep disruptors have been introduced into mainstream media. If you are having sleep challenges, it behooves you to evaluate the impact that these factors may have on you.

Ambience

Better sleep comes with a dark, cool, and quiet room. Light signals to the brain that it is day time and stimulates a cascade of hormones to boost your energy. As part of your natural circadian rhythm, your body temperature naturally drops as night approaches, signaling to your brain that it's time to slow down and get some rest. When you keep your bedroom cooler, it reinforces your body's natural instinct to sleep. A warm environment makes it more difficult to fall asleep. Noise keeps your mind alert and can cause difficulty in falling asleep and cause you to wake up throughout the night.

Blackout shades or an eye mask can foster a dark, cozy environment. Ear plugs can dampen a bed mate's snoring or residual house sounds. These items, in particular, have been crucial in assisting me to get some great quality sleep. Honestly, I procrastinated for many years before surrendering to ear plugs and an eye mask. I encourage you to take action now and learn from my experience.

I used to love sleeping with my window open for the cool air. But I found that I spent a lot of hours during the night listening to what was happening outside my bedroom window. I lived in the forest with acres surrounding the house, but even so there was a lot of activity happening outside. I could hear raccoons, deer, frogs, the wind, rain, trees creaking, and even my cats passing in and out through the cat door. Obviously, I was not sleeping. Hence, the ear plugs!

Peace. Quiet. Darkness.

Blue Light

Blue light comes from our TV, phone, iPad, computer, LED, and video games.

Blue light is part of the natural visual light spectrum, since it is part of sunlight and it is energy efficient, so it has become the popular option for lighting. This efficiency is bolstered by the removal of red light. In nature blue and red light always coexist and play a vital role in controlling our circadian rhythm.

This is why you probably sleep better on nights when you have spent the day outside in the sunshine. However, exposure to blue light at night confuses our natural cycle, stimulating the brain to think it is still daytime. Not ideal when you need to get some Zzzz.

Yet, blue light is commonplace in our homes: we watch TV, surf the internet, get consumed with social media, read, and game on our devices right up until we expect to fall asleep. This is a significant and common cause of sleep problems, including insufficient and low-quality sleep. This exposure affects our performance on many levels from cognitive performance, learning, and memory to physical performance, allostatic load, and energy levels.

Not only does exposure to blue light have negative hormonal consequences, it also has damaging effects to our mitochondria. Blue light causes a breakdown in mitochondria, inhibiting their performance, increasing the production of ROS, and accelerating cell death. We have already linked mitochondrial dysfunction to chronic degenerative diseases, cardiometabolic disease, obesity, neurodegenerative disease, and others.

Mitochondrial health is required for our survival. Compromised performance leads to aging and disease. Focusing on increasing mitochondrial performance will help us to not only heal, but also to thrive.

You should avoid blue light for at least two–three hours prior to going to bed. Keep your lights dim. Adjust your screens to emit warmer and dimmer light if you are continuing to use your devices. Blue blocking glasses are another way that you can help to protect your mitochondria.

EMF

EMF are found in smart phones, wireless internet, anything with voltage, electric clock radios, power meters, power lines, cell towers, microwaves, and even hair dryers.

Electromagnetic fields are not visible, so we often don't realize we are being exposed. Unfortunately, EMF are everywhere, and as wireless technology advances, our exposure continues to increase. And even if you are not aware that it is happening, they can affect the electrical communication in your body. Brain waves, nerve transmission, and cell-to-cell communication can all be affected.

EMF exposure can cause symptoms of sleep disruption, mood swings, and headaches. It has also been correlated with increased ROS, cancer, neurodegenerative disorders, and reproductive challenges. We have already discussed the vicious cycle of mitochondrial dysfunction and the resulting increase in ROS production which leads to more mitochondrial dysfunction and more ROS production, etc. This oxidative stress adds to your allostatic load.

It is virtually impossible to avoid exposure, unless you are living off the grid! However, you can make an effort to reduce your exposure by charging your devices away from the bedroom. Only use your laptop and other devices on battery, not while they are charging. And I know you have heard it before, but do not sleep with your phone on by your bed unless it is off (and not charging) or on airplane mode (and not charging).

Apnea

Sleep apnea is very common in people with cardiovascular disease and with obesity. This breathing disorder is associated with episodes of intermittent hypoxia, oxidative stress, sympathetic activation, and endothelial dysfunction, all of which are critical mediators of cardiovascular disease. It is also associated with metabolic syndrome and insulin resistance.

Normal sleep provides a time of low physiological stress and increased parasympathetic nervous system activity. Apnea causes an increase in physiologic stress and increases sympathetic activity, oxidative stress, and inflammation, so instead of a calm period of rest and recovery, you are in a heightened state of fight or flight. This does not make for a very productive sleep and can result in fatigue, brain fog, and hormone dysregulation.

Many people do not even know that they have sleep apnea. It is usually diagnosed following a sleep study. However, the American Alliance for Healthy Sleep has indicated common symptoms of sleep apnea to include:

- Loud or frequent snoring
- Silent pauses in breathing
- Choking or gasping sounds
- Daytime sleepiness or fatigue
- Unrefreshing sleep
- Insomnia

- Morning headaches
- Waking during the night to go to the bathroom
- Difficulty concentrating
- Memory loss
- Decreased sexual drive
- Irritability

Sleep apnea not only increases your own allostatic load, it increases your bed mate's as well. Continuous positive airway pressure (CPAP) therapy is a common treatment for sleep apnea. However, avoiding alcohol, performing moderate exercise, and maintaining an optimal BMI can help to improve the symptoms of sleep apnea and your sleep quality.

Pets

This is a touchy subject for me because I did let my 100 lb. rescue dog sleep on my bed. And he was a big sleep disruptor, literally. But now that he has passed on (RIP good boy), my stance and recommendation is "no pets in bed," or in the bedroom for that matter. I guess we will see how strong that stance is if and when I get another pup to love.

Honestly, you need to remove and limit any of the factors that can compromise the quantity and quality of your sleep. Pets often snore and are restless, and often times they are not on the same sleep schedule as you, waking up during the night or in the early hours before dawn. In addition, if you are prone to allergies, a pet in bed can elevate your exposure and symptoms.

Optimize Your Zzzz

How much sleep do we really need? That depends on you. Evidence supports needing seven–ten hours of sleep per night, depending on your age and where you are on the health continuum. I said sleep, not lying in bed tossing and turning. Quality of sleep matters more than quantity in this regard.

A study at Emory University found that individuals who reported six or fewer hours of sleep had higher levels of inflammatory markers, the basis for disease. Sleep increases both health and vitality. More than twenty large scale epidemiological studies all report the same clear relationship: the shorter your sleep, the shorter your life.

For the cynics out there, sleeping excessively will not bring more health and vitality. The sweet spot seems to be in the 6.5- to 8-hour range. In my experience with my patients, people who are challenged with pain or active disease processes require more sleep since they are expending a tremendous amount of energy on healing and repair (much like how children require more sleep to support their rapid rate of brain and body growth and development).

The Oura ring can be of great assistance when it comes to dissecting your slept patterns and quality. It has been a game-changer for me. I was able to see objectively how a restless night resulted in a higher resting heart rate and poor recovery. A few nights of minimal deep sleep translated into major fatigue and brain fog for me, even though I was "sleeping" eight hours per night. Quality matters. The Oura ring takes the guesswork out of my bio-hacking. And while it does a fantastic job of collecting data and showing trends, it does not do the actual work of creating proper sleep habits.

Good Sleep Hygiene

Have a Nightly Ritual

This will help to alert your brain to prepare for sleep and helps to build a strong sleep hygiene habit for improving the quality of your Zzzz.

It works well to go to bed and get up in the morning at about the same time every day. Strive to be asleep before 11:00 p.m. to avoid a cortisol burst that can keep you up long into the night. Think of it as a second wind. Wake up by 7:00 a.m. every morning, and try to avoid falling back to sleep once light has hit your eyes. This initial light exposure triggers the burst of cortisol that has been building during the night to give you that boost you need to get you moving and out of bed.

My nightly ritual looks something like this.
An hour before bed, I take an Epsom salt bath infused with lavender and eucalyptus oil. During this bath, I read, or I listen to binaural beats. After the bath, I complete the following:

- Make sure to rinse off with warm, clean water before drying off
- Apply coconut oil to my face and body
- Brush and floss my teeth
- Prepare my water for first morning consumption
- Crawl into bed and do my gratitude journaling and snuggle

Nest

Your mattress and bedding can make all the difference in providing you the physical space to surrender to your delta waves. Keep your choices organic and free of chemicals. Parachute is a fan favorite for bedding on many levels, including quality of product, eco-consciousness, and philanthropic mindset. Having a cozy and comfortable bed makes you look forward to the time you will be spending there.

Clear the clutter

Your bedroom is for sleeping and making love. Not work. Clutter raises stress and reminds you of all the things you need to deal with, which is bad timing when you are attempting to calm down and relax.

Tone it down

You want the environment to be cool, dark, and quiet. Use eye shades and ear plugs if you must. Take precautionary measures to feel safe and secure so that you can surrender to sleep.

Practice Insights

- Plan your sleep habits. Go to bed at the same time and wake up at the same time every day.
- Strive for eight hours of **quality** sleep every night.
- Ditch the disruptors.
- Invest in an Oura ring if you are serious about stress, sleep, and performance. Check out my website for more information and a link to purchase at www.drnancymiggins.com.

Practice 6: Move

Let's Up Our Game

We have become a sedentary society with the vast majority of people sitting inside in front of computer screens every day, all day. An astonishing 80 percent of Americans do not get the recommended amount of daily exercise! This lack of movement takes its toll on the spine, joints, ligaments, muscles, and fascia. Not to mention, it can lead to hormone imbalance and depression.

We have all experienced the burst of motivation that happens in January to "get in shape." However, this motivation fades relatively quickly, and the desired results are rarely obtained or sustained.

This is because the focus is most often on vanity. Don't get me wrong; everyone wants to look their best. However, rock hard abs and a super lean body cannot be achieved in a few hours, weeks, months, or maybe ever—especially if you are stressed out, tired, dehydrated, or undernourished.

I am going to interchange the term movement with exercise because I hope to inspire a perspective change—a paradigm shift, if you will, designed to increase your level of success when it comes to exercise. This unconventional approach will help us achieve and maintain a healthy body. Rather than focusing on vanity, we are going to focus on healthy. Health happens on a cellular level and is driven by the performance of your mitochondria. Movement creates the momentum to shift your trajectory away from disease and redirect it to favor health instead. The change happens on the inside first, microscopically, before you realize an increase in your energy level and before you can build a lean and toned body. Optimal mitochondrial performance is healthy. Healthy is sexy. Healthy is beautiful.

It is important to become healthier and increase movement. Please understand the long-term implications of you and your children spending hours in front of a screen working or playing games, rather than being outside playing games that require movement. Being physically active is the most significant and protective habit to reduce cardiometabolic risk and obesity. This applies not only to you, but also your children and grandchildren. They learn by your example.

Your relationship with exercise is built early in life. I was fortunate to grow up in a fairly remote place. My family did not experience the pressure of technology consumerism. Parents in our neighborhood sent kids outside to play, every day, rain or shine, even on the harshest winter days when it was far below zero on the thermometer. We would gather to play kick the can, boot hockey, baseball, or some other made up game. We worked in the garden, helped carry and stack firewood, shoveled snow, mowed the lawn, and were asked to help out however and wherever we could.

It was not that long ago that physical labor was an important part of daily life and survival. Past generations worked much harder for much less. They didn't have to go to a gym or specifically train for physical fitness since it was a by-product of life.

In recent decades, the exercise movement has exploded with many exercise gurus. One such guru was Jack LaLanne, an early health innovator and a physical fitness inspiration icon. And you may not know this, but he was also a chiropractor. While he did not personally practice the art of chiropractic, he did apply the science and philosophy to his daily life and used this as the basis for the instruction he gave his many loyal fans.

He built an empire, inspiring households with his calisthenics and dietary advice. Jack LaLanne pioneered the fitness movement and paved the way for the multitude of innovators, gyms, and personal trainers that have continued to expand the industry over the past seven decades.

The principles that Jack LaLanne shared when he first aired in the 1950s still hold true today. While we have updated terminology and methods, the core principles are the same.

Today, there are probably as many exercise theories as there are diet theories. Some of the training programs have worked for some people. However, most of them have not worked for most people in the long run. The methods and requirements are not sustainable by the masses.

Movement goes beyond building muscle or aerobic capacity, although these are important side effects of exercise that can help increase your vitality and expand your health span. We are all aware of how moderate exercise can reduce the risk of cardiovascular disease and obesity. We know that individuals who engage in regular exercise and physical activity have significantly lower rates of disability and an average life expectancy approximately seven years longer than their sedentary counterparts. And active people enjoy a much longer health span.

Lack of Movement

Movement is the cerebrospinal fluid pump circulating this fluid within your central nervous system. Cerebrospinal fluid protects the brain and spinal cord, acting as a shock absorber. It bathes the brain with vital nutrients and helps to eliminate toxins.

Movement works to balance brain hemisphere activity and stimulates neurotransmitter and hormone production, leading to improved mood and cognitive function. There is a consistent association between higher levels of physical activity with greater volume of the prefrontal cortex and hippocampus in older adults. These are the areas that tend to decline in adulthood and that support executive and memory functions. Incorporating daily movement into your life can be an effective prevention for cognitive impairment and other behavioral problems associated with brain atrophy.

Your brain is not the only thing that can waste away with age. Your muscles tend to do the same. Sarcopenia, an age-related condition resulting in muscle wasting and weakness, is one of the most important causes of functional decline and loss of independence in older adults.

Beginning as early as our forties, evidence suggests that our muscle mass and muscle strength decline in a linear fashion, with up to 50 percent of our developed muscle mass being lost by the time we reach our eighties according to an article published in Current Opinion in Rheumatology in 2012. Obesity and fat infiltration into the muscle accelerate this degeneration.

There are many factors that contribute to sarcopenia, including the obvious decline in activity level and nutrition, as well as an increase in generalized inflammation. But mitochondrial performance is at the center of this degenerative and progressive condition. It is vitally important to foster the optimization of mitochondrial function to support and maintain muscle. It gets harder and harder for us to build and keep muscle as we age.

Too Much of a Good Thing

Is there really such a thing as too much exercise? Recent evidence suggests that a "tipping point" may exist whereby too much exercise becomes detrimental to the cardiovascular system and your health.

When we engage our muscles in any type of exercise, we place an increased demand on the mitochondria, requiring more ATP to fuel our body. ROS is a by-product of ATP production, and so increased activity also increases ROS levels. We have talked extensively about the effects that this has throughout your body over time.

Within your cardiovascular system, ROS contribute to endothelial dysfunction; think of this as leaky gut of your blood vessels during extreme exercise. Intense bouts of exercise elevate systolic blood pressure and cause inflammation of the blood vessels promoting an oxidative environment. Oxidative stress contributes to endothelial dysfunction. Over time, this can lead to atherosclerosis, hypertension, diabetes, and chronic heart failure.

Now calm down, I am not promoting that exercise is bad. However, over-exercise and excessive training can have unexpected and dire consequences, especially when there isn't ample time for your body to recover and heal the damage, and if you do not have ample antioxidants to neutralize the ROS before they cause any long-term damage to your cells and body as a whole. The goal is to find the delicate balance that exploits the benefits of exercise while minimizing the taxing effects on your body.

There is no one-size-fits-all when it comes to an exercise program. Each of us has unique needs and considerations that play into what elements will provide us with the best sustainable results. Obviously, a deconditioned or diseased person may not be able to enjoy the same level of activity as someone who is relatively healthy and has incorporated movement consistently in their life. It will take some time to build the strength, flexibility, and endurance required to live a healthy and active lifestyle.

Ultimately to improve your level of function and endurance, you have to know where you are starting from and build from there. You should not expect to go from a desk jockey to an ironman competitor in an instant. It requires systematic training and intermittent healing to develop the stamina to complete any endurance event. Basically, you need to walk before you can run.

Start with Your Heart

I know, I know, you want a sexy beach body. Who doesn't! But if you don't handle what is happening on the inside of your body, you will never achieve the results on the outside. Healthy is what we are going for. Sustainability is what we are striving for.

It is time to get intentional. The quality of your movement is more important than the quantity. Moreover, consistency is crucial to success.

If you aren't measuring and monitoring, then you are guessing. It is easy to rationalize (rational lies) your efforts and performance unless you are tracking, which provides you with objective feedback from your body. So let your body dictate how much and how often you should move, not an exercise plan or training regime.

Your ultimate bio-hack is to find the balance of sufficient movement and sufficient rest and recovery. Heart rate variability is a great indicator to identify and track the appropriate level of activity.

There are five different heart rate training zones. These zones are defined as percentages of your maximum heart rate. We each have an individual resting heart rate and maximum heart rate. While the percentages that define heart rate zones are standard, the actual heart rates will be unique to each person.

Resting Heart Rate

You learned how to determine your resting heart rate in practice 4. This is an important metric for you to know and monitor when living an active lifestyle, especially if you are upgrading your movement habits. As you recall, you want your resting heart rate to be sixty beats per minute or less.

If your resting heart rate falls above that level, this indicates you are not recovering from stress efficiently and are experiencing allostatic overload; thus, you need to start slow and build some cardiac endurance before increasing your exercise duration and intensity. You will want to pay close attention to your heart rate training zones. Slow and steady will be your mantra.

Having a resting heart rate within the desired range means that you are ready to jump in with both feet. However, even a 5 percent increase in your resting heart rate indicates that you have not recovered fully and need to enjoy a rest day. Keep your activity limited to a leisurely thirty-minute walk, nothing more. As soon as your resting heart rate is within normal again, you can increase your exercise and intensity.

How to Measure Your Resting Heart Rate

While we discussed how to measure this in practice 4, it also applies here, so here are the instructions again. Your resting heart rate is an important number to know and monitor. To determine your resting heart rate, measure your pulse first thing in the morning before getting out of bed. Do this several mornings in a row to get an average.

You can determine your resting heart rate by locating the pulse in your wrist and counting the beats for ten seconds, then multiplying this number by six. Ideally you want your resting heart rate to fall between sixty–sixty-five beats per minute, or less.

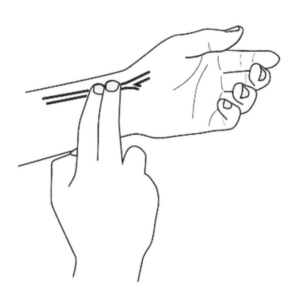

Remember that you want to increase your vagal dominance. If your resting heart rate is high, you have low vagal activity and your sympathetic nervous system is calling the shots, namely stress. You will want to start slow and be patient. Love and nurture yourself along the way so you will be able to enjoy the benefits of your efforts for the long haul.

It is important to track your resting heart rate daily. It is a good indication of how your body is responding to exercise and recovering from the exertion. If your resting heart rate is elevated even by 5 percent, you need a rest day. Not a light workout day, a rest day.

How to Determine Your Maximum Heart Rate

It is easy to determine your age-predicted maximum heart rate. This is the highest heart rate you can safely hit during exercise.

220 minus your age = max heart rate

Your max heart rate decreases with age. You can see how that math works in your favor. You will be able to achieve your desired zone exertion with much less effort as you age because your zone thresholds will be lower.

Using a heart rate monitor and keeping your level of effort less than 70 percent of your maximum heart rate is the ideal place to start. Technology, such as the Fitbit, calculates your maximum heart rate and tracks how much time you spend in a particular training zone.

Whether you go old school or new school on tracking, it is very important to know your numbers and track them consistently. This will dramatically improve your efficiency and results.

Training Zones
Zone 1: Very Light
50–60 percent of maximum heart rate
Training in this zone will help to improve your exercise recovery rate. Walking is a perfect choice for this zone because you can easily control your pace to keep your heart rate within the zone.
Zone 2: Light
60–70 percent of maximum heart rate
Training in this zone helps to improve your endurance and metabolism and muscle strength. Walking and yoga are great options.
Zone 3: Moderate
70–80 percent of maximum heart rate
This improves blood circulation.
High intensity interval training (HIIT)
Zone 4: Hard
80–90 percent of maximum heart rate
Breathe hard, aerobic training, increase speed endurance
HIIT
Zone 5: Maximum
90–100 percent of maximum heart rate
Your heart and lungs will be working at their max. It is difficult to sustain efforts at this level.
Do not attempt to train at this level.

Optimize Your Intentional Movement

Creating a healthy body and expanding your health span does not require a gym membership or fancy equipment. You were blessed with all the tools you need when you were born.

Just think of all the money I just saved you! You can invest it in organic food to fuel your body and optimize your mitochondria.

Aerobic

Your daily minimum goal is to walk five miles or about ten thousand steps in zone 1. Walking in nature expands your benefits exponentially: Breathing fresh air, encountering a variety of surfaces and terrain, and absorbing natural light add sensory complexity to your walk. Meeting other walkers, and their dogs, creates an opportunity for you to have social interactions and connection.

Additionally to meet your aerobic needs, you could go dancing, running, rowing, swimming, or cycling. However, I like to keep things simple, and walking doesn't require anything fancy. The gravitational stress helps to strengthen your bones without the jarring effects on your joints that comes with running. Rowing, swimming, and cycling do not give you the same bone health benefits as walking.

Get off the treadmill. Grab a friend, or your dog, and walk. It is simple, highly underrated, and incredibly effective.

Resistance

As part of creating and maintaining health, it is important to build a strong, lean body. The older we get, the harder it is to keep our muscle strength and mass. Let alone build muscle. Regardless of your age, you need to start today. And don't stop.

The idea that you have to spend endless hours at the gym is outdated. Developing a healthy, fit body and keeping it does not require working harder, longer, or more frequently. It is about working smarter.

HIIT, is the optimal way to boost mitochondrial biogenesis. That's right, intense bouts of exercise stimulate your mitochondria to increase in size and to replicate, thus increasing your potential energy output. Numerous studies have demonstrated that mitochondria increased by 25–35 percent after six to seven sessions of HIIT. To achieve maximum results with HIIT, you need to allow for ample rest so only do this a maximum of three times per week. Give yourself a day or two of rest in between.

To meet your HIIT needs, you can do a series of body weight exercises that can be done anywhere without any special equipment. These exercises are designed to give you the biggest bang for your effort buck. They will help you develop strength and coordination as a solid foundation to build on. Once you have established a strong foundation, you have many options to up the ante and diversify your program.

Be honest with yourself about your starting point. This includes acknowledging your present or past injuries, current level of fitness and agility, and current strength. Start slow and be smart. It is always wise to consult your primary care physician when embarking on a new exercise regime.

Be real and celebrate your authenticity. This is not the time to compare yourself with others; simply start from where you are at and build from there. If you do this, you will reduce your risk of injury and setbacks. This simple program is designed for the long haul.

One Set of Each

25 SQUATS

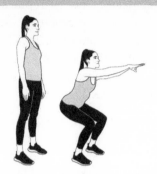

25 LUNGES
EACH LEG

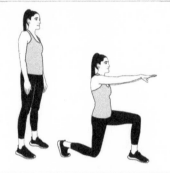

25 CRUNCHES

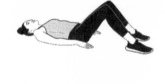

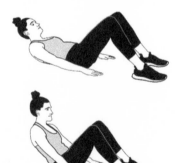

15 PUSH-UPS	
25 SUPERMAN BACK EXTENSIONS	
1-MINUTE PLANK	

Start with one set three times per week. Work your way up to four sets three times per week. In total this should not take you more than twenty minutes to complete. Alternatively, you can do four individual sets spaced throughout the day; just make sure that you allow for a minimum of two hours between sets to maximize the benefits. Keep your pace up, breathe in and out through your nose, keep your mouth closed, and remember to hydrate between sets. Try to avoid resting between sets if you are doing multiple sets in a row.

According to a study published in the *International Journal of Exercise Science* in 2017, nitric oxide production increased twofold with nose breathing as compared to mouth breathing during exercise. While exercising, you need to ensure that oxygen gets to the cells for energy production by the mitochondria since nitric oxide dilates blood vessels. The blood vessel dilation will help to escort metabolic by-products, like lactic acid, out of the muscle tissue. You can avoid some muscle soreness with nose breathing.

If you cannot do fifteen traditional push-ups, I suggest you start with "modified" push-ups and keep your knees on the floor. Continue to start each set with traditional push-ups and then revert to the easier version as soon as you lose good form. One good form push-up will quickly turn into two, and eventually you will be completing all four sets of fifteen.

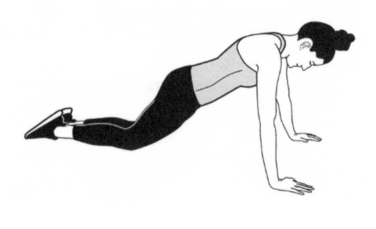

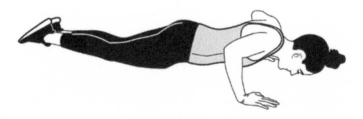

Form is essential, and I will say it again: quality is more important than quantity. You will never build a solid foundation if you continually compensate for your weakness; you want to rewire your nervous system and build muscle memory. Start slow and build slowly to avoid reinforcing negative movement patterns. Even if you can only do five proper crunches, you will get more benefit from those five than by doing twenty-five poor form ones.

There is no shame if you have to use a chair or the wall to support your balance when you start to do squats and lunges, especially if you haven't done these in a while (or never). It is possible that you may lack the strength and flexibility required to do a full squat or lunge. If this is the case, use support and be patient with yourself. The strength and flexibility will come with time and consistency.

It is important to track your progress. There will be days when your motivation is waning and you will question whether the effort you are putting in and the pain you are going through are actually making a difference. This is where your journal will come in handy. You will be able to quickly recognize your successes and identify where you may need to put some extra effect or focus.

Flexibility

Yoga is a practice that involves physical movement, strengthening and stretching activities, focused breathing, mindfulness, and meditation all wrapped into one. Yoga promotes movement within the ability of the individual, enhanced body awareness, and self-compassion. It has the potential to help people of different shapes and sizes feel comfortable with movement and activities that increase strength and flexibility, which can lead to sustained physical activity over time. And that is what we are going for: movement habits that can be incorporated into daily life and sustained for a lifetime.

We discussed in practice 4 how yoga helps to increase vagal dominance and decrease stress and allostatic load. It is the combination of mind body relaxation techniques along with mild to moderate physical exercise that optimizes our innate anti-inflammatory mechanisms which help to prevent oxidative stress and promote a healthy immune response.

Yoga has many different types of practices, and I recommend that you experiment and find the one(s) that work for you, and then incorporate yoga into your daily routine, at a minimum of four days per week on days that you do not do HIIT.

A dear friend of mine introduced me to the Down Dog app when I was traveling frequently for work. I struggled to maintain consistency with my movement habits because I was traveling at least two weeks out of each month. Down Dog provides daily yoga practice options that can be catered to the individual, allowing you to select the difficulty and duration so you can easily adapt it to your schedule. It costs less per year than two yoga classes at a studio. I love it for its flexibility, no pun intended.

Circadian Rhythm

Because your muscles have an internal clock just like your brain, your exercise efforts can yield different results depending on what time of day you are performing them.

Certainly, your life schedule will dictate, in a large part, what your movement routine will look like. However, I have found that morning and midafternoon are preferred over evening exercise for your HIIT or power yoga.

Exercising in the morning has many benefits. Morning exercise makes it easy to exercise while fasting, which will amplify the benefits you receive. The combination of fasting and exercising maximizes the impact of cellular factors that force the breakdown of fat and glycogen for energy. Training on an empty stomach will effectively force your body to burn fat, which is useful for preventing both weight gain and insulin resistance. In addition, morning movement helps to reduce food cravings and increases your tendency to up your total activity level during the day. It essentially puts you in the right mindset for your success.

Midafternoon has its upside as well. It helps to offset that afternoon energy slump that typically happens around 2:00 p.m. Opting to do some movement may help prevent you from self-medicating with sugar, junk food, or caffeine.

Evening is a great time for yoga or a walk. These activities activate the parasympathetic nervous system and help you to calm down and relax. This can aid in better sleep, which synergistically helps to lower stress.

If you work a sedentary job, it is important to take mini-breaks to facilitate hydration and movement. Get up and do some stretches or squats, go for a lap around the office, or step outside into natural air and sunlight for a few minutes and walk around the block. Your productivity will go up as a result of these self-love acts of kindness.

Again, there is no one right answer. The important factors are quality of movement and consistency. Your consistency on a daily and weekly basis will help to support your circadian rhythm for both exercise and sleep. You need to move every day. We all do.

Practice Insights

- Create a daily and weekly schedule to incorporate intentional movement into your routine. Daily walking, yoga, and three sessions a week of HIIT will provide incredible, life-changing results.
- Keep your movement efforts within the desired heart rate training zone for the activity. More is not necessarily better.
- Track your movement and results.

Practice 7: Purify

Personal Responsibility to Yourself, Your Children and the Planet

The saying "think globally, act locally" is deeply ingrained in this section. We are naïve to think that air pollution in one region of our country or world does not impact the air quality of the entire planet. The same goes for water pollution and the ripple effect that it has on the quality of our drinking water and quality of our agriculture that relies so heavily on irrigation for crops and water for livestock. All water is connected.

Because of our negligence in these areas, we are now seeing huge health consequences. We are amidst a chronic inflammatory disease epidemic. It is alarming how fast the rate of disease, in general, is accelerating in our country.

Environmentally Acquired Illness (EAI) refers to a variety of serious chronic health problems caused by exposure to mold, pesticides, heavy metals, air pollution, dust, and other irritants found in the environment. EAI is fast becoming a common issue, presenting in clinics and practices of all types.

As you recall, inflammation is one of the three responses to stress. In this chapter I focus on chemical stress. And while the focus is on this one stressor category, remember that stress in all its forms ultimately translates to inflammation, oxidative stress, and immune dysfunction as the means for the body to combat the stressor. The repercussions of chronic stress on these innate healing mechanisms results in cardiometabolic disease, neurodegenerative disease, autoimmune disease, and cancer.

We need to wise up! The only way to change the rate of degradation of our planet—and ultimately our health—is to vote with our dollars. We have the influence and power as consumers to change the current status quo. Stop supporting the companies, industries, and governments that do nothing to inhibit the onslaught of toxins.

Toxic Burden

In this day and age, there is no way to ensure that you are breathing clean air, drinking clean water, or eating clean food. Even if you grow your own food or purchase only organic products, you are still exposed to a variety of toxins or toxic residue. We have contaminated all of our resources. I know, the truth hurts.

According to an article published in *National Geographic* magazine, each year the US Environmental Protection Agency reviews an average of 1,700 new compounds that industry is seeking to introduce. Yet the 1976 Toxic Substances Control Act requires that they be tested for any ill effects before approval only if evidence of potential harm exists. This is seldom the case for new chemicals. The agency approves about 90 percent of the new compounds without restrictions. Only a quarter of the 82,000 chemicals in use in the US have ever been tested for toxicity, according to the article.

To shed some light on the magnitude of this problem and hopefully inspire you to make some different choices, I will highlight some categories of toxics (note that there are more than these). If enough people start to make positive choices, it will have a large enough financial impact on the few key companies that are in control. Those consumer driven industries will be forced to make changes in an effort to maintain their market share and continue to reap financial rewards.

These are the key health disruptors and their impact on your health is growing.

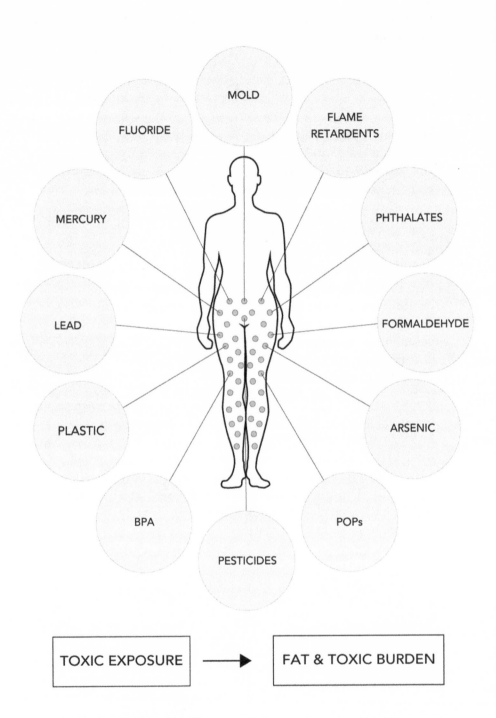

Heavy Metals

Heavy metals are not biodegradable. They are persistent environmental contaminants and can be present in air, water, soil, food, and dust. These exist as natural substances in nature, meaning they are not man-made.

The Agency for Toxic Substances and Disease Registry (ATSDR) publishes a priority list every two years. This list identifies substances that have been determined to pose the most significant threat to human health due to their known or suspected toxicity and likelihood of exposure. The top three substances on the 2017 list are all heavy metals.

Arsenic

This substance is found primarily in pressure-treated wood used for decks and outdoor playsets prior to 2003. Arsenic compounds are also used in pesticides and as an additive in animal feed.

Rice and rice products contain high levels of arsenic. While rice and other plants grow, they absorb arsenic from the soil and water. Consumer reports published a couple of articles on the subject, and the FDA has now issued what it considers to be safe levels of consumption. You can monitor their findings on the FDA.gov website.

As we identified in the chapter on hydration, arsenic is commonly found in ground water. If you are on a well, you should have your water tested. All municipalities are required to provide a detailed water report for consumers purchasing city water. Know what you are drinking.

Lead

Lead and lead alloys are commonly found in pipes, storage batteries, weights, shotshells and ammunition, cable covers, and sheets used to shield us from radiation during x-ray or other diagnostic imaging. Lead compounds are used as a pigment in paints, dyes, and ceramic glazes. It is often present in caulk.

The largest source of lead released into our environment was through leaded gasoline exhaust. Unfortunately, this fuel was not completely banned until 1996.

There is *no* safe level of lead consumption. Let's not forget the 2014 water debacle in Flint, Michigan. That tragedy is a reminder to us all that we need to pay attention and take action. We cannot assume that anyone else has our best interest at heart.

Mercury

This substance has a few different forms in nature. Generally, mercury is used in production of chlorine gas and caustic soda, and in extracting gold from ore. Dental fillings typically contain about 50 percent metallic mercury. It is also used in thermometers, barometers, batteries, fluorescent light bulbs, and electrical switches.

Mercury is an extremely toxic substance and every caution should be taken if a thermometer or fluorescent light bulb breaks in your home. The EPA and the ATSDR have detailed instructions on how to clean it up. Following these instructions will limit your immediate exposure, as well as long-term repeated exposure.

Mercury compounds have been used as fungicides, topical antiseptics, disinfectant agents, and skin-lightening creams.

Not only do we encounter it in products, but it can also be in what we eat as it accumulates in fish. Species of fish that are high on the food chain and typically have longer life spans, such as tuna, shark, swordfish, and sturgeon, tend to have higher levels of mercury. Pescatarians should be mindful of the type of fish they are consuming, as well as the quantity.

Other common heavy metals that negatively impact our health are cadmium and aluminum. Cadmium exposure is especially high in smokers, while aluminum is ever present in deodorants and antiperspirants.

Heavy metals disrupt metabolic functions in two ways: they accumulate in vital organs and glands—such as the heart, brain, kidneys, bone, liver, reproductive system, and fat—and they displace the vital nutritional minerals from their binding sites. This inactivates or modulates critical enzyme systems and protein structures leading to cellular dysfunction and disrepair.

Over time being exposed to heavy metals causes them to excessively accumulate in the body, producing free radicals, both ROS, and reactive nitrogen species. This leads to oxidative stress. The unifying factor in determining toxicity and carcinogenicity for all these metals is the generation of reactive oxygen and nitrogen species.

Plastic

We live in a plastic world. It is everywhere and it is going to be here forever because it is convenient. But this convenience factor compromises your health and your health span.

According to a study published by the Royal Society of London in 2009, approximately 4 percent of world oil production is used to make plastics. A comparable amount is used for energy in the production process. It is disappointing to say the least that over a third of the current production of plastic is used to make items of packaging, which are then rapidly discarded.

It is not sustainable to continue to dedicate our dwindling fossil fuel resources in this way. We are already feeling the environmental impact from our overflowing landfills and massive oceanic flotsams.

This affects you and your family in a more profound way than you may realize. Research demonstrates that a mixture of plastic-derived compounds, BPA and phthalates, can promote epigenetic transgenerational inheritance of adult onset disease. In this 2013 study published in the peer reviewed journal *PLoS One*, researchers found that when gestating ancestors (great-grandmothers) were exposed to these plastic compounds, their third generation offspring inherited their adult onset diseases and obesity.

This is a big deal! Here are just a few of the more common components in products that we use every day.

Bisphenol-A (BPA)

BPA is used to make polycarbonate plastic and epoxy resins which are in turn used in a variety of plastic items such as water bottles, sports equipment, medical and dental devices, dental fillings and sealants, household electronics, and eyeglass lenses. It is also used in the receipts you get from most merchants, including the grocery store, gas station, and restaurants. BPA is an endocrine disruptor with widespread exposure and multiple adverse effects, including impaired reproductive capacity, promotion of obesity, and metabolic disease.

Bis (2-ethylhexyl) Phthalate (DEHP)

DEHP is widely used as a plasticizer in manufacturing articles made of polyvinyl and plastic bottles. It is considered a reproductive and developmental toxicant.

Dibutyl Phthalate (DBP)

DBP, a phthalate used primarily as a plasticizer to add flexibility to plastics, is used as a component in latex adhesives, cosmetics, and cellulose plastics, and as a solvent for dyes.

Phthalates are commonly found in personal care products. Recent studies suggest that some phthalates can alter human male reproductive development.

Since infants are commonly exposed to lotion, powder, and shampoo, they experience widespread exposure as confirmed in 2008 in *Pediatrics*. Researchers found that 80 percent of babies screened were exposed to measurable levels of at least nine different phthalate metabolites.

Pesticides

Pesticides include compounds labeled as insecticides, rodenticides, herbicides, fungicides and fumigants. These are highly resistant to environmental degradation.

Like other substances discussed above, pesticide exposure and its resultant oxidative stress response can lead to a variety of disease processes and dampen your health span. And like plastics, pesticides can promote epigenetic transgenerational inheritance of adult onset disease.

Probably the most prolifically used pesticide in history is the controversial herbicide Roundup, which Monsanto introduced to the public market in 1974.

Roundup was not selective; it killed every plant it came in contact with. So in 1994 Monsanto introduced its first genetically engineered crop, Roundup Ready Canola, which was planted in 1996.

Basically, Monsanto found a solution (herbicide) that created a bigger problem (improper application would jeopardize crops) for them to solve. They solved it by creating genetically modified organisms (seeds) that were Roundup resistant, allowing farmers to spray the herbicide without damaging their crop.

Most often when you mess with Mother Nature, she kicks you in the ass. In March 2015 the World Health Organization's International Agency for Research on Cancer concluded that glyphosate, the active ingredient in Roundup, is "probably carcinogenic to humans."

In 2017 the European Union voted in support of phasing out glyphosate over the next five years in all twenty-eight countries. They immediately banned household use.

There have been hundreds of suits filed against Monsanto. Last year, jurors awarded $289 million to a man who developed non-Hodgkin's Lymphoma from repeated Roundup exposure.

Genetically engineered crops with tolerance to glyphosate are widely grown, and their use has led to the increased application of glyphosate. This is found not only in our food, but also in our water. Worldwide, glyphosate contaminates drinking water via rainwater, surface runoff, and leaching into groundwater, thereby adding drinking water, bathing, and washing water as possible routine exposure pathways.

The emergence and spread of glyphosate-resistant weeds requires farmers to spray additional herbicides, including older herbicides posing documented environmental and public health risks. This sounds a lot like how bacteria have evolved with the introduction of antibiotics. Nature is amazing!

For decades Roundup was considered safe. Its perceived nontoxicity was predicated on the assumption that our cells do not possess the shikimate pathway, a biological pathway in plants, which is disrupted by glyphosate.

However, our gut bacteria do have the shikimate pathway. We depend upon this pathway in our gut bacteria, as well as in plants, to supply us with essential amino acids. Many hormones and neurotransmitters depend on the shikimate pathway metabolites as precursors.

Chronic exposure to glyphosate provokes oxidative damage by disrupting mitochondrial metabolism through increased production of ROS. The effects are most commonly realized in the liver and kidneys. However, glyphosate is highly neurotoxic, posing a threat to the brain and nervous system.

It is also a chelating agent with the potential to sequester essential micronutrients that are required for the multitude of enzymatic activities that occur within the body. As a chelator, it can also influence and facilitate the uptake of arsenic and aluminum—both of which are known toxins.

Persistent Organic Pollutants (POPs)

POPs are a group of highly toxic chemicals that include the insecticide dichlorodiphenyltrichloroethane (DDT), poly-chlorinated biphenyl compounds (PCBs), and industrial waste products such as dioxins. These chemicals were widely used after World War II until the United Nations treaty the Stockholm Convention was signed in 2001 which blacklisted the twelve most detrimental chemicals. Since that time continued efforts have been made to eliminate or restrict the production and use of POPs.

However, POPs are very slow to degrade, and they are known to accumulate and pass from one species to the next through the food chain. So we can be exposed by eating contaminated animals or being exposed to the pollutant in the air. Upon exposure, the body works to confine the toxins in fat tissue. While this helps to preserve the liver, kidneys, and brain in the short term, these accumulated POPs are slowly released into the bloodstream. Weight loss triggers an increase in the level of circulating POPs within your body.

Interestingly enough, POPs are obesogenic. They cause you to gain weight as you create more fat to store and sequester the toxins. It becomes a vicious cycle which increases systemic inflammation and ultimately disrupts metabolic function.

While these chemicals are banned, new formulas are created. POPs are commonly used as flame retardants and water repellants in clothing, as pesticides, and as a means to help control mosquitos in malaria-prone areas. And they are commonly found in waste products of industry being purged into the air and water.

According to the World Health Organization (WHO), more than 90 percent of human exposure to POPs is through food, mainly meat and dairy products, fish and shellfish. Even low levels of POPs can lead to increased cancer risk, reproductive disorders, immune system dysfunction, neurologic impairment, endocrine disruption, DNA damage, and increased birth defects.

Mold

Not all mold is bad. Consider mushrooms, wine, beer, and cheese. Mold and fungus are everywhere, inside and out. On a recent trip to Minnesota, I was surprised to see so many people experiencing "allergies" when there was still snow on the ground. Seasonal allergies are usually associated with spring time and the increased pollen counts coupled with budding trees. Since trees are still dormant in northern Minnesota in March, mold was the culprit for this surge of allergy symptoms, more specifically snow mold.

Snow mold is a fungus that damages grass as the snow melts. You would think that the extreme temperatures would kill the mold; however, it can go dormant. Snow mold can cause allergy-like symptoms. Again, mold is everywhere, whether you know it is there or not.

While we can't control snow and external environments, we can control inside our homes. It is estimated that about 50 percent of homes have mold growing. The trouble with mold is that often times you don't even know it is there. It can be odorless, but at times there can be a musty or toxic odor.

It is virtually impossible to eliminate all mold and mold spores from within your home. The way to control indoor mold is to control moisture. Bathrooms, basements, and attics are common areas for mold to grow; thus, it is important to fix leaky faucets, windows, and roofs before mold can take root.

Exposure to mold and mold spores can happen immediately or may be delayed, and this exposure can trigger inflammatory reactions, oxidative stress, and immune responses. Chronic mold exposures can induce infection, toxicity, allergy, respiratory compromise, autoimmune disorders, mitochondrial toxicity, kidney toxicity, and neurotoxicity, and DNA damage.

Patients often present with a chronic inflammatory response syndrome, also known as CIRS.

They complain of broad symptoms including fatigue, brain fog, muscle and joint pain, insomnia, depression, and anxiety. The development of new onset chemical sensitivity is also commonly seen after exposure.

Research has shown that none of the commonly used methods for cleaning water-damaged materials such as bleach, ammonia, ultraviolet (UV) light, heating, and ozone were found to completely remove mold and mycotoxins from water-damaged building materials. In cases of severe exposure or reaction, it may be necessary to vacate the premises and find a new home.

It is important to avoid further exposure to contaminated items such as clothing, stuffed animals, furniture, and carpets. In addition, you should make every effort to decrease exposure to other chemical agents including pesticides, heavy metals, cleaning products, fragrances, vinyl chloride, plastics, nonstick cookware, and other toxins in an effort to reduce the total toxic load being placed on the body.

Mold also grows on food. It grows on everything. If you are particularly sensitive to mold, it is best to avoid bread, cheese, mushrooms, nuts, and berries because they have a high affinity to mold. Also, beer, wine, fruit juice, and hard cider should be avoided.

One of my patients, a middle grade school teacher who taught cooking, had a chronic exposure to black mold. Her classroom was one of several newly constructed annex buildings.

She had been under my care for several months over her summer break. When school started in the fall, she began to experience a wide array of symptoms that did not make sense to her. She became extremely tired and fatigued, although she had difficulty sleeping. She complained of brain fog and random migrating joint pain and developed multiple food sensitivities. She actually felt as though she was sensitive to *everything*: light, food, noise, smells, and touch.

It took some detective work, but we eventually figured out that her symptoms got worse when she was in her classroom. Black mold was identified within the walls.

Once the stressor was removed, she could start the healing process. It took her a good two years before she felt "normal" again. This is how powerful toxic exposure can be and how deeply complex the manifestation of exposure is.

Compounding Interest

Many illnesses may be caused or exacerbated by a person's exposure to environmental toxins. These include, but are not limited to Alzheimer's disease, dementia, Parkinson's, autism, autoimmune diseases, cancer, Type II Diabetes, metabolic syndrome, obesity, leaky gut syndrome, asthma, and allergies.

Often times these environmental toxins can have a synergistic effect. While exposure to one substance may not result in an overt physical or physiologic response, exposure to multiple toxins can magnify the response exponentially.

Patients often claim they don't have a negative reaction to any of the above items. Unfortunately, it is not a matter of "if," it is a matter of "when."

Lack of a profound reaction does not mean that your body was not affected. It only means that your body successfully sequestered or eliminated the toxin.

Your body will work to detoxify and protect you the best it can. But all of these toxic substances accumulate over time and cause damage. Just because you have not been diagnosed with diabetes or cancer today, it doesn't mean that you are not knocking on that door.

Remember, it takes time to build disease just as it takes time to build health. Your body is in a constant battle trying to overcome disease and dysfunction while preserving health. The more that you expose yourself to these toxic substances, the more bioaccumulation and adverse effects your body experiences. And one day it will not win the battle.

Strategies to Mitigate the Toxins

It is overwhelming when you consider the daily onslaught of toxic exposure that we endure. With knowledge comes the power to make different choices and inspire positive change so our children and our children's children can enjoy a different reality and a longer health span.

Every choice matters. Small changes combined with other small changes can have a huge impact over time.

To take control over your environment and reduce your toxic burden, follow the three steps below. (It is important to maintain some perspective here because you are not likely to eliminate everything.)

1. **Remove** toxic substances from your home.

Evaluate all of your personal and home care supplies. This can be a very daunting experience, so I suggest you start with personal care items. Tackle home care and cleaning products next. Finally, address your yard care products.

Your body won't release your current toxic load if it is continuing to be poisoned every day.

2. **Replace** these items with clean alternatives. The EWG is a great resource to identify good products for your home and personal care.

Try to simplify and reduce the number of products you use. For example, coconut oil has countless uses including body lotion, shaving cream, makeup remover, face moisturizer, personal lubricant, hair conditioner, and homemade deodorant. It can also be used to pull oil for good oral health, to cook, and to use as a source of healthy fat and medium-chain triglycerides.

3. Repair and rebalance your body. Incorporate the other seven practices into your daily life to support your body and give it what it needs. It will do the rest.

Optimize Your Purification with
These Daily Detox Rituals:

Drink warm lemon water

This stimulates the liver and digestion and helps to purge toxins that have built up over night

Oil pulling

Swishing coconut oil around in your mouth for ten minutes prior to brushing your teeth helps to decrease bacteria, plaque, and gum inflammation. Coconut oil has antibacterial and antifungal properties. Spit the oil out into trash; don't swallow it.

Tongue scraping

This helps to promote good oral hygiene and reduces bad breath by removing bacteria and mucous that contains toxins.

Dry brushing

This stimulates circulation, lymphatic drainage, and exfoliation. Brush from your hands and feet toward your heart using a natural bristle, long handled brush. Do this before your shower and then moisturize with coconut oil after.

Epsom salt detox bath

Add two cups of Epsom salts, one cup of baking soda, and ten drops of lavender to your bath. The magnesium and lavender will help you sleep (an important part of supporting detox) and the sulfates help the body get rid of toxins.

Hot yoga/infrared sauna

Sweat it out! Your skin is a huge organ of detoxification.

- Vote with your dollars.
- Eat organic.
- Protect yourself and your loved ones by restricting exposure to known toxins.
- Create a habit of daily detox.

Practice 8: Gratitude

Wired for Success

The idea that having a mindset of gratitude will somehow improve your health and extend your health span may be hard to grasp. However, neuroscience actually backs this up. We can be wired for success.

It was once believed that the brain you were born with was the brain you had for life, and it could not be altered. This hypothesis has long been replaced with the phenomenon of neural plasticity.

Neurons and brain cells have the ability to adapt their structure and function in response to what is happening inside your body and in your environment. Only those neurons that are connected to your immediate experience through your senses and emotions will fire. In addition, new neural connections will start to form within minutes. The more connected the neurons, the stronger, more responsive, and more effective that area of the brain will be.

Neural plasticity is this mechanism by which the brain and nervous system encodes experiences and learns new behaviors. We actually grow new nerve fibers and produce denser nerve networks through a process called arborization. Think of it like a tree expanding its branches or root system to support its growth.

Likewise, the brain and nervous system is continually pruning to cut back areas where there is little activity or stimulation. The neurons that aren't as needed will eventually wither away. Since we don't want our body to waste precious energy or resources maintaining a highly energy dependent but dormant tissue, this withering away is normal and healthy. This is one way the brain grows into its most efficient self.

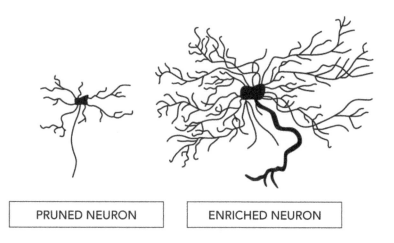

| PRUNED NEURON | ENRICHED NEURON |

This process of pruning and natural selection happens continuously and innately by design. What we put our focus toward tends to expand our awareness and activation of the particular neural network that supports that stimulus. The brain and nervous system, like every other system and cell of the body, seeks efficiency. Repetition reinforces a pathway and increases its efficiency. Emotion in conjunction with repetition synergizes the effect. Use it and improve it.

Think about when you learned to drive a car. At first you had to consciously manage all of the micro-tasks involved. You had to think about keeping your hands in the right position on the steering wheel, pressing on the gas pedal, checking your rearview mirror, and using your signals. You learned to manage all of these things during high emotional states, including excitement, fear, uncertainty, and joy.

Fast forward six months. Now you are driving in rush hour, putting on your makeup, chewing gum, and talking on the phone without any conscious consideration to the management of the multitude of tasks and skills required to drive. Obviously, this is not the best strategy for avoiding an accident or a ticket. However, it does provide a good visual for how your brain and nervous system can adapt and grow from experiences, repetition, and practice.

On the other end of the spectrum, let's say you learned to speak French in high school. In this situation you are not completely immersed in the culture; you are only exposed for a few hours a day for a few years.

Fast forward to your midlife crisis and your trip to Paris. It is likely that your brain has let the pathways that were developed in high school dwindle. Since your neural networks were not actively engaged in speaking French for an extended period of time, those networks degraded and you are no longer fluent. Use it or lose it.

Power of Optimism

Your mindset, emotions, and experiences all play a role in how your brain evolves and grows. Every time we have an experience, the corresponding neural network is activated. Every time it is activated, the neural network gains greater importance. Repeating or prolonging an experience will keep the connections between neurons strong and ensure they stay viable.

This is of critical importance to understand. Your mindset and emotions, both positive and negative, have a major effect on the structuring and functioning of your brain.

According to the National Science Foundation, 80 percent of our daily thoughts are negative and 95 percent of those thoughts are repetitive thoughts. Many of these thoughts and perceptions make up our internal map of reality, which was formed in childhood. These thoughts occur outside of our present time consciousness; it is like they are an automatic reflex. This does not set us up for success, especially when trying to make lifestyle changes. The magnitude of this negative thinking paralyzes us and prohibits consistent change in our behavior and choices, making it near impossible to create new habits.

Negativity elevates the stress response and all of the implications it has in the body. As you recall, stress has a profound effect on heart rate variability and mitochondrial performance, and ultimately our allostatic load. We know that heart rate variability and mitochondrial performance are markers of biologic aging. Their efficiency reflects our resiliency, essentially our ability to adapt effectively to stress and environmental demands.

Therefore, your mindset can largely determine the efficiency of your brain function. Brain neurons are rich in mitochondria. Each neuron contains about two thousand mitochondria, while the rest of the body averages two hundred mitochondria per cell. The brain is the most metabolically active organ in the body and is very vulnerable to disruption of energy resources, including that of mitochondrial dysfunction. Disturbances in brain energy metabolisms lead to disease, ranging from subtle alterations in neuronal function to cell death and neurodegeneration, and can manifest as brain fog, dementia, Alzheimer's disease, and Parkinson's.

The brain is our most critical organ, and mitochondrial health is at the center of brain health. Mitochondria are particularly sensitive to stress. Regardless of the source, stress has been associated with lower mitochondrial energy production capacity. The brain and nervous system control and coordinate all of the activities and functions happening within your body. Compromising the mitochondria in the brain compromises everything. This should reinforce the importance of incorporating all eight practices outlined in this book into your daily life.

Give your brain and body what it needs and eliminate what it doesn't. No part of us "needs," or even wants, negativity. Even if it seems like your brain feeds on it. Research at the HeartMath Institute confirms that one of the most powerful factors that affect our heart rate variability is our feelings and emotions. This is important because we know that heart rate variability is a predictor of mortality. Meaning, low heart rate variability, indicating a high stress load, shortens your life span and your health span. In addition, research published in 2018 in *Biological Psychology* identified that a negative mood, especially at night, was related to lower mitochondrial performance and energy output which increased the allostatic load on the body.

A mind that is rooted in shame, worry, fear, self-criticism, and guilt creates a brain and nervous system that supports pessimism, worry, anxiety, and depression. This neurology holds you hostage and keeps you paralyzed from following through with positive choices by constantly bringing negativity to your awareness.

Relax, this is not a death sentence, and you are not doomed to live in negativity forever. In the same way that you can create a brain rooted in pessimism, you can redirect your neurology to support positivity. Remember, what we put our focus toward tends to expand our awareness and activation of the particular neural network that supports that stimulus.

Focus on positive feelings and work to put a positive spin on situations and experiences. Your brain will adapt to reflect this new pattern. It will strengthen neuronal connections that support resilience, gratitude, and self-esteem. As you become deeply rooted in optimism and positivity, your stress level and allostatic load will decrease.

For instance, it is easy to become negative and resentful when you are constantly cleaning up after your children, doing laundry and dishes, cooking meals, and going grocery shopping. This part of parenting is a thankless job, and an endless one. It is easy to feel as though you and your efforts are being taken for granted. However, you can re-posture your feelings to be those of satisfaction and fulfillment. You can be grateful for the opportunity to take care of your family and your ability to do so at the highest level.

When you combine positive emotions and conscious optimism, you will grow neural networks associated with this mindset. This new, calm state will give you grace under pressure. It will help to create an environment where your mitochondria can thrive.

Conscious Appreciation

There is a formula for success when it comes to rewiring your brain. Many methods and approaches, like positive affirmations, neurolinguistics, reading, and meditation may help to get you there. The Holosync technology that was discussed in practice 4 is a great adjunct in helping to reinforce positive brain wiring. Certainly, employ any and all of these that you have interest in or time for. It comes down to consistency, repetition, and emotion.

I like to keep things simple and efficient. Expressing thanks and gratitude in writing is as simple as it gets. Again, simple does not mean easy—at least in the beginning.

Like any other habit or skill, gratitude takes practice to be developed. It requires an appreciation of the positive aspects of your life. It should not be a comparison to someone else's situation, good or bad. This is your opportunity to shine light on the things that matter in your life, big or small.

An attitude of gratitude can change everything in your life for the better. Attitudes inspire thoughts and emotions. Thoughts and emotions determine behavior. Your behavior determines your actions. Those actions determine your results. And ultimately, it comes full circle: your results influence your attitude, which can help to modify your internal map of reality.

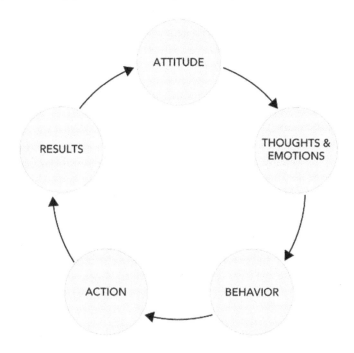

When we think about what we appreciate, the parasympathetic or calming part of the nervous system is triggered. That influence can have profound and protective benefits on the body, including reducing our allostatic load. Cultivating a feeling of appreciation has been shown to reduce the stress hormone, cortisol, by 23 percent. In addition, it increases coherence in heart rate variability patterns, resulting in vagal dominance and a balanced and responsive HPA axis. People with an attitude of gratitude experience lower levels of stress.

Gratitude has also been implicated in benefits ranging from better physical health and enhanced immunity and self-esteem to improved sleep and a reduction in the effects of aging on the brain. At this point you are well-versed in the role that mitochondrial performance plays in health and disease and the implications that stress and allostatic overload have mitochondrial function. Instead of the popular phrase of "happy wife, happy life," it should read "happy mitochondria, happy life"! Never mind. It doesn't rhyme. With a practice of gratitude, you can look forward to fewer aches and pains, a sharper memory, and restful sleep.

Gratitude reduces social comparisons. Grateful people are able to appreciate other people's accomplishments, as well as their own. It fosters an "equal and different" perspective rather than one of comparison or envy. This mindset is a healthy way to support yourself and others and can be incredibly helpful when embarking on a new healthy lifestyle. Celebrating the small, daily achievements helps you to stay motivated to continue your progress day after day.

Gratitude begets gratitude. The feeling of gratitude increases activity and blood flow to the hypothalamus in the brain, which is located in the midbrain and plays a vital role in motivation. This is where our thirst instinct and hunger instinct are located. The hypothalamus is also responsible for governing the autonomic nervous system and determining whether the sympathetic or parasympathetic nervous system will be engaged at any given time and it rules the endocrine system. So you can see why the boost in activity and blood flow associated with the feeling of gratitude would be beneficial in your overall well-being. Gratitude stimulates a chemical cascade of hormones and neurotransmitters, including:

Dopamine

Dopamine "feels good," and is often associated with reward, pleasure, and satisfaction. It triggers a reward cascade and inspires action. A spike in dopamine makes you more likely to do the thing you just did. Therefore, once you have the feel-good benefits of gratitude, you'll want to keep feeling it.

Oxytocin

Oxytocin is the "love drug" hormone. Your feelings of gratitude can actually increase the bond and intimacy you feel toward your partner, family, and friends. Boosts in oxytocin is a very good thing. It will give you even more reasons to be grateful!

Serotonin

Serotonin has been called the "happy" chemical. Moreover, unlike dopamine's quick fix, serotonin creates a state of contentment which has a much longer lasting effect. People who enjoy life tend to experience a longer health span. Gratitude leads to a sustainable form of happiness. It is not based on immediate gratification; it is a frame of mind. Don't worry, be happy.

There is obviously an abundance of benefits, both emotional and physical, to gratitude. Another great attribute is that gratitude costs absolutely nothing to practice. Anyone can be grateful for their life and make the practice of gratitude a daily habit.

By practicing gratitude daily, you will see a ripple effect throughout your life. The rewiring of your brain and nervous system may take a while to grab hold; however, the pay it forward impact within your sphere of influence happens immediately. You will see the change in your spouse, friends, coworkers, and children. In no time at all, you will have inspired a subtle shift of consciousness. It is contagious. Everyone in your daily life will be expressing more appreciation and gratitude, resulting in a greater and greater number of positive inputs into your nervous system. This will snowball into broader branches and deeper roots of optimism within your brain. And you can see how the cycle continues as your stress decreases and your health improves.

Throughout this book we have talked about many downward spirals and the negative effects of vicious cycles on your mitochondrial performance, your overall allostatic load, and your health and health span. Finally, with the practice of gratitude, we have a positive vicious cycle and upward spiral!

Optimize your Gratitude

Think it and ink it. I have been very blessed in my life to have had many exceptional mentors and coaches. Throughout all of their messages, it has been clear that one should physically write down both their goals and what they are thankful for—and review them both often. There are no shortcuts to success here.

An important part of the intention and emotion around the practice of gratitude is generated with the power of the pen (or pencil). Keeping a gratitude journal ingrains the process on a deeper level, both emotionally and neurologically. It helps to make gratitude part of our life experience.

Initially, it may be somewhat difficult to identify what you are grateful for. I know it was for me. When I first started this practice, I had weeks of being grateful for my children, a good night's sleep, and my dog. I didn't expand on any of these things. I kept each one short and simple, just a word or two. But initially, those were the only things that I could think of as I stared at the blank page.

My writer's block caused many questions, more accurately concerns, to run through my mind: Is that all I really had to be thankful for? I guess I really do need this on a daily basis. Does everyone else have this much trouble? What is wrong with me? This is not helpful right now; it only makes me feel worse. My frustration grew on a daily basis, but I continued my commitment to practice gratitude every day.

And then one day I wrote down "a beautiful sunrise." A few days later I penned "a warm embrace." My entries expanded in concert with my awareness. Suddenly, and yet so subtly, I found myself being grateful for things like a chance encounter with an old friend; a sunny day amidst a gray, wet Seattle winter; a stranger opening the door for me; close friendships; a random passerby complimenting me on my smile; and the list went on. I became aware of the multitude of senses, feelings, and experiences that inspired me on a daily basis.

The little things in life suddenly carried great meaning for me. The warm cup of coffee, made with love and intention, that was delivered to me in bed along with a gentle kiss on my forehead was now an exceptional life experience rather than a beckoning to get my ass out of bed.

You get the picture. What you focus on expands. As I consciously looked for reasons to be grateful and appreciative, miraculously I found them! My brain now seeks them with little effort from me. Gratitude is a mindset.

In addition to memorializing the things that I am grateful for each evening, I also set an intention each morning to identify ways that I would make each a great day. This is not a task list or prioritized to-dos. It is a grounding and focus on what I will bring to the table and how I will interact with the world to make it a better place. This was also a practice in frustration when I first started.

It seemed that every day was the same. I had no variety. I apparently had no spice in life! Lead with grace and compassion, drink water, walk, and love my dog were my daily mantras. Don't get me wrong, I felt fulfilled every day. I just lacked the awareness that would expand myself and my success.

But again, as I persevered, the words, and the actions to support those words, came. I got very clear on how I wanted to show up in my life every day, how I could have a positive impact on those around me, and what I needed to do for myself to be my best self, for me and for others. My performance improved and so did my efficiency. I had a clear path to walk and it minimized distractions.

Once I identified what was needed for me and from me, I started to feel bad if I did not accomplish "my list of attributes" or live up to my goal. I was getting swallowed up in shame and self-defeat. This negativity creeping in was undermining me, eroding my optimism, and challenging my commitment. It is amazing the stronghold that negativity has in our lives and over our lives.

I bring this up because I don't want you to despair or allow yourself to get derailed when you experience this. It is not a moral defect. It is not a fault of your willpower or determination. Instead, see it for what it is—old thought patterns. The key word being old. You are working to create a new mindset and a new thought pattern focused on gratitude and optimism. Love yourself and persevere.

In an effort to keep this in check, I added another component of journaling every evening. I started to write down what I could have done better or different and I acknowledged where I was struggling or was not living up to my potential. This alleviated the burden of my self-imposed expectations. And by writing it down, that mental chatter did not keep me up at night. I was not mulling it over throughout the night when I was supposed to be sleeping. I was no longer a victim to it.

This process helped to attract and cultivate success in my life. I was being wired to attract what I wanted. And I became more content with my life as it is. Not complacent, but content. Thank you, serotonin!

The daily practice of gratitude can change your life. I know it did mine.

Practice Insights

- Set an intention with actions to support it.
- Acknowledge successes and failures.
- Express appreciation and gratitude.

Part 3: Personalizing Your Health Strategy

"Let go of who you think you're supposed to be;
embrace who you are."

—Brene Brown

Hopefully, now that you have made it to the final section of this book, you haven't decided to toss these practices aside because it all sounds like way too much work. It is work. A lot of work for the rest of your life. Your life depends on it!

You are responsible for your health and health potential. You are responsible to lead and guide your children to adopt healthier habits. I hope you are not still thinking that our current health care system or social security program will provide you with an actual health outcome. These programs have finite resources and a primary goal of profitability, not helping you achieve your desired health outcomes. And try as we might to find answers to solve our current and growing health crisis, insurance programs are not the answer.

Through the current health care system, our doctors can only treat and manage disease; they are not managing your wellness. For the most part, they have no control, no authority, and no answer for preventing people from realizing chronic degenerative diseases, like diabetes, heart disease, obesity, Alzheimer's disease, and cancer in the first place. In addition, they have no cure.

Doctors are frustrated by the current state of affairs; it is not just patients. Many want to help people. They have dedicated at least a decade and hundreds of thousands of dollars to education for the primary goal of helping people and making a difference in the world. However, since they can't always achieve that within traditional primary care settings, many are leaving and seeking training in alternative and functional medicine disciplines so they can offer solutions outside of the insurance-driven paradigm.

It is not acute, crisis care, such as treatment for trauma and broken bones, that is bankrupting the system. It is the management of these chronic degenerative diseases with no cure that is growing our debt load as fast, if not faster, then our waistlines. We may be living longer than our ancestors, but we are not really "living" in our advanced years. We are just dying for a longer period of time.

The *New England Journal of Medicine* published a special report titled "A Potential Decline in Life Expectancy in the United States in the 21st Century" in 2005. The article not only identified obesity, and its related disease complications, as the primary factor in our longevity reduction, it also made clear that the youth of today may, on average, live less healthy and possibly even shorter lives than their parents.

Prevention has been a buzzword in the world of medicine for many decades. Prevention within the medical paradigm is focused on screenings for early detection of a disease process that can lead to early intervention and treatment. While this has provided benefits, it still lacks the important aspect of providing tools, support, and education to promote personal responsibility in lifestyle choices to avoid disease. There needs to be a much broader community involvement to support healthy living. A good example of this took place in Finland. The Bulletin of the WHO published an article in 1998 revealing the effects that lifestyle modifications had on Finland's cardiovascular disease mortality rate. In 1972 Finland had the world's highest cardiovascular disease mortality rate. To combat this, an active community-based prevention program was implemented countrywide that included healthier food options and anti-smoking legislation. They used a variety of ways to educate the public, including media, schools, worksites, and spokespersons from sports, education, and agriculture. They did not see immediate results; however, within five years significant improvement in smoking, cholesterol, and blood pressure were documented. In just over twenty years, Finland has reduced their cardiovascular disease mortality rate by 75 percent, as well as reducing all causes of mortality. This is an impressive endeavor. Just think about how much more efficient a campaign like this would be today with the use of modern technology.

Unfortunately, we are still operating a grassroots campaign in this country. Big Pharma has the loudest voice and deepest pockets, but we can change that as each of us, one by one, adjusts our diet and lifestyle. The practices in this book are designed to help you take control over your health and minimize your risk of disease. They are tools to extend your health span, not just your life span. Disease is not your destiny.

Mindset

It all starts with making a choice, a decision, and a commitment to change. Change is not easy. It is not comfortable. At times it can even be painful, both physically and emotionally. Most often, however, positive change is worth the discomfort, especially since it is usually short-lived. In fact, the majority of our suffering happens in our mind when we are contemplating change, even before we take our first step into action.

Do not let fear and uncertainty win again over your desire for a better life. Now is the time to be bold and lean in. You are the number one priority in your life. You deserve to be your best. If you are not performing at your best, everything in your life suffers as a result. When you are less than your optimal self, it not only affects you, it also affects your relationships. Give yourself permission to take control of your health. You have everything you need within you to succeed.

Metrics

The practices in this book contained a variety of measurements detailed to assist you in identifying your starting point. You need to know where you are starting from so you can create a personal health strategy to reach your goals. But just know, a starting point is just that, a point in time. It becomes quickly irrelevant if you do not take action.

Periodic reassessment of these key measurements allows you to see tangible improvements as you take action implementing and sustaining the eight practices. You will also feel your success as your energy and sleep improve, your excess pounds melt away, and your thoughts become clearer and more focused as you reduce your exposure to common toxins and liberate those toxins that have accumulated over your lifetime. Happiness and contentment will be hardwired into your brain through gratitude and feeding your body what it needs and eliminating what is doesn't.

Tracking and reassessing these metrics will help you to stay the course. Often times the magnitude of change that you desire seems overwhelming and unattainable. Break it down into manageable steps with realistic goals. Just let each step and success motivate you to take one more step. You are comparing you to you, no one else. You are not competing with anyone else, but you may be racing against the clock depending on your age and where you are located on the health continuum.

Below you will find a list of all the metrics and the instructions of how to calculate each one. There are a few bonus metrics that were not discussed previously in the book. If you are serious about taking control, I strongly suggest that you go the extra mile to obtain all of these baseline measurements and record them. Revisit these measurements monthly (blood work every six to twelve months) to evaluate your progress.

Hydration

It is difficult to measure hydration within your body. However, you can measure and document the amount of water you consume on a daily basis. Write down your current intake before you start the thirst challenge, then document your daily water intake thereafter.

After successfully completing the ten-day thirst challenge and re-establishing your thirst instinct, strive to consume at least half of your body weight in ounces of water every day. You may find that you are thirsty for more, drink it and document the amount.

pH

Over the years my patients have struggled with testing their pH for the first time. The uncertainty stems from the testing process feeling too "science-y." Relax, if you mess up the process on one day, try again the next.

Get yourself some pH strips. A roll will cost you under ten dollars and last you a very long time. Using a two-inch piece, dip a test strip into first morning urine. You can either collect urine in a cup or attempt to pee directly onto the strip. I use a cup. Dip a separate two-inch piece into first morning saliva. I use a spoon to collect saliva and then dip the test strip into it. Avoid putting the test stripe into your mouth. You should not drink water or brush your teeth prior to collecting your urine and saliva, just get out of bed and measure first thing.

The test strips will have a color code to match your strip to a corresponding pH value. Try to color match within thirty seconds for the most accurate reading. Salivary pH tends to be more alkaline, while urinary pH will tend to stay in the acidic range.

Use the following equation: **2x salivary + urinary ÷ 3 = pH.**

Do this for three mornings in a row, then record your average pH. Use this average as your starting pH value. Your pH value should be greater than 6.3.

Body Measurements

At a minimum you will want to measure your height and your waist and hip circumference. Record your height in feet and inches, for example 5'9". Record each circumference in inches.

This is an important metric, not for aesthetic reasons—although inches are often lost even when weight is not, when incorporating the eight practices—but because a high waist circumference is associated with an increased risk for type 2 diabetes, dyslipidemia, hypertension, and cardiovascular disease. To minimize risk for these diseases, women should keep their waistline less than thirty-five inches and men should keep their waistline less than forty inches.

Waist-to-hip ratio is commonly used as a metric to assess risk for the same diseases. Calculate your waist-hip ratio using the following equation: waist inches ÷ hip inches = w-h ratio

Acceptable ratios are less than .85 for women and less than .90 for men.

Weight

Weigh yourself first thing in the morning after you urinate. Be naked, no shame. Write down your weight. Remember to weigh yourself under the same conditions when you remeasure your weight.

I don't use weight as a determinant in the success or failure of a health-driven program. Typically, weight fluctuates on a daily basis. A little monosodium glutamate (MSG), a very common food additive, can cause a 10 lb. weight increase due to its cellular disruption and water retention effects. In addition, increasing lean muscle mass through proper movement as described in practice six can also stymie weight loss on a scale. Your metabolism will increase with more lean muscle and more mitochondria in your muscle cells. Often people will lose inches and drop clothes sizes, even though their weight on the scale has not changed.

Body Mass Index (BMI)

This considers a ratio of your height to your weight. Doctors and personal trainers often use this metric as a marker for health. However, it does not take into account your body composition specifically because it is not a measure of lean muscle mass. Your BMI will change with every pound that you gain or lose. However, it is a good tracking metric and guidelines have been established to help you determine whether you fall within the optimal range.

> **To calculate your BMI, use the following US National Institutes of Health three-step equation or one of the many options online:**
> weight in pounds X 704.5 = #
> # ÷ height in inches = #2
> #2 ÷ height in inches = BMI

A BMI of 18.5–25 is considered normal. If you fall between 25–30, you are overweight. If you exceed a BMI of 30, you are considered obese.

Blood Pressure

Blood pressure is another useful metric to monitor your health over time, but it is influenced by diet, exercise, medications, and stress. To get the most accurate reading, measure your blood pressure first thing in the morning prior to eating, drinking, or exercising. If you don't have your own blood pressure cuff, most pharmacies offer free blood pressure screening. A normal blood pressure is considered to be 120/80 or below. My "sick" patients have trended high with their blood pressure, while healthier patients trended below normal. Most everyone can reduce their blood pressure naturally by following the eight practices consistently.

Resting Heart Rate

Your resting heart rate needs to be measured first thing in the morning before you even get out of bed. Find the pulse in your wrist or your neck. Count the number of beats for ten seconds and multiply this number by six. This gives you the number of heart beats per minute. Ideally, you want this number to be sixty beats per minute, or less.

Maximum Heart Rate

You will want to determine your maximum heart rate. This is a key number in determining your heart rate training zone limits.

Use this equation: 220 − your age = max heart rate. Record the number.

Record this number and use it to calculate your heart rate for each type of movement you are doing. You will want to stay below 70 percent of your maximum heart rate for most activities, like walking and yoga. You will want to be at 80 percent of your maximum heart rate when doing your HIIT.

	Day1	Day 30	Day 60	Day 90	Month 6	Month 9	1 Year
Hydration (oz)							
pH							
Height							
Waist							
Waist to Hip Ratio							
Weight							
BMI							
Blood Pressure							
Resting Heart Rate							
Maximum Heart Rate							

Blood Work

It is important for you to know your blood lab numbers. If you haven't had your blood checked in a while, now might be a good time to get some baseline numbers. While there are endless tests that can be done to check everything from vitamin D, hormones, neurotransmitters, and food allergies and sensitivities, at this point we can keep things simple and get just some core tests done. These tests in particular will help to identify risk for cardiometabolic disease. I included optimal values in the chart. Note that "optimal" does not necessarily mean "normal" range. You are striving for optimal.

Contact your primary care doctor to inquire about getting these tests done. It is not uncommon to have them performed as part of an annual physical. If you have results for these tests that were obtained within the past twelve months, you can use them as your baseline.

These tests are typically included in regular blood work:

Triglycerides

Total Cholesterol

HDL

LDL

C Reactive Protein

Hemoglobin A1C

Fasting Insulin

Fasting Glucose

I am including the following chart to make it easy for you to track your success and metrics, as well as your goals. It is also available on my website: www.drnancymiggins.com

	Optimal	Day 1	Month 6	1 Year
Triglycerides	<100			
Total Cholesterol	<200			
HDL	>50			
LDL	<100			
C Reactive Protein	<1			
Hemoglobin A1C	<5.2			
Fasting Insulin	<3			
Fasting Glucose	<85			

Strategies for Success

There are a few key strategies that will help you to succeed. Whether you find yourself in a position of just needing to fine tune your habits and do a minor course correction, or you are in dire need of a diet and lifestyle makeover to inspire a dramatic shift in your health trajectory, systems and processes can help to keep you focused and efficient in your efforts.

Starting any new endeavor can be intimidating, and sometimes even overwhelming. Hopefully, these strategies will help to ease this transition for you.

No Plan is a Plan Destined to Fail

Planning and being prepared is critical to your success. This sample calendar shows how you can schedule your self-care for the week. Obviously, I do not know your specific schedule so this is just an idea of what a week of daily rituals might look like.

You will need to customize a schedule for yourself. The important part is to have a schedule so that you can keep *you* as the priority and schedule everything else around you.

Monday	Tuesday	Wednesday	Thursday	Friday	Saturday	Sunday
Hydrate first thing and throughout the day	Hydrate first thing and throughout the day	Hydrate first thing and throughout the day	Hydrate first thing and throughout the day	Hydrate first thing and throughout the day	Hydrate first thing and throughout the day	Hydrate first thing and throughout the day
morning sun salutation yoga	morning walk	green drink	morning walk	morning sun salutation yoga	Green drink	Green drink
green drink	green drink	Lunch time HIIT	green drink	green drink	morning yoga	long walk
lunch time HIIT	lunch time binaural beats	evening walk	lunch time binaural beats	lunch time HIIT	long walk	evening restorative yoga
evening walk	evening hot yoga	dry brush	evening hot yoga	evening walk	dry brush	gratitude journal
dry brush	gratitude journal	Epsom salt bath (binaural beats)	gratitude journal	gratitude journal	Epsom salt bath (binaural beats)	
Epsom salt bath (binaural beats)		Gratitude journal			Gratitude journal	
Gratitude journal						

Engage

Most every successful endeavor requires a support system. You need encouragement, so don't be afraid to be vulnerable and ask for support. You can lean on your partner, a friend, or group of friends. It is human nature to not want to disappoint the people we care about. Pick your support system wisely, however, because whomever you surround yourself with will need to be your biggest cheerleader. In the end, you are leading this endeavor and you will ultimately need to have a strong will in addition to their supportive influence. You have the power and control to determine your health.

Success is much sweeter when we have people to share it with. Writing down and sharing your goals will help keep you accountable to them. Failure on any given day is not failure of you or the program. There is no shame in failure, only shame in the lack of attempt or lack of taking action in the first place. I have named each element a "practice" for that very reason. You practice them every day.

Make sure to acknowledge and celebrate your victories, large and small. The people who love and care about you will be thrilled to be on this journey with you.

Detox Your Pantry

I have found over the many years that I have worked with patients that this is a touchy subject. There really is no easy answer.

If your house and pantry is stocked with food you should avoid in order to build health, then you need to get rid of them. Just like an alcoholic shouldn't hang out in a bar, you are more likely to slip if you see those items every day no matter how strong-willed and committed you are.

It is best to pack up all of the processed food and junk food and donate them to a local food bank. The following chart may help you to sort through your cupboards and purge those items that will not serve you or your health, or your family's health for that matter.

Refined Beverages	Eliminate all soda (even diet), fruit juices, milk, soy milk and any sweetened milk alternative including hemp, rice or almond. Also purge flavored water that uses sweetener and artificial colors, flavors or preservatives.
Packaged Foods	This includes items like chips, cookies, crackers, boxed cereals, salad dressing, candy, sweets and other refined foods. Even if it says "healthy" or "low fat" on the box - purge it.
Processed Cheese Products	These are highly processed and full of artificial food dyes, taste enhancers, saturated fat, and partially hydrogenated oils.
Cured Meats, Sausages, Lunch Meats, Hotdogs	These meats contain nitrites, preservatives, saturated fats, and sodium.
Margarine, Lard, Shortening	The hydrogenated oils and trans fats increase toxicity in the body.
Commercial White Bread and Baked Goods	These products are made with refined flour and are typically high in sugar with little nutritional value.
Conventional Dairy Products	The acid-forming nature of dairy, along with hormones, antibiotics and other toxins present can cause inflammation in the body. These include milk, yogurt, sour cream, cream cheese, cottage cheese, cheese, and ice cream.

Plan Your Food

People often ask, "How in the world do I eat ten servings of vegetables every day?" The answer is simple: plan.

In practice 3 we discussed the importance of promoting a more alkaline pH. This is accomplished largely by eating more vegetables and eating less food that produces acidity. I have seen time and time again that the body can heal many disease processes, and promote health, when appropriately nourished.

I am including an example menu to show you how easy it is to get your ten servings of vegetables and two servings of fruit each day. Remember to keep your food consumption restricted to an eight- to ten-hour period and avoid eating three hours prior to going to bed.

Example Menu

Day 1	Day 2
16 oz. water 1 cup of hot lemon water enhanced with raw apple cider vinegar and cayenne pepper Green drink	16 oz. water 1 cup of hot lemon water enhanced with raw apple cider vinegar and cayenne pepper Green drink
Bulletproof style coffee or tea (1 tablespoon coconut oil and 1 tablespoon grass-fed butter)	Bulletproof style coffee or tea (1 tablespoon coconut oil and 1 tablespoon grass-fed butter)
Mixed greens salad avocado, cucumber, shredded carrot, tomato, shredded beet, hard-boiled egg Balsamic dressing	Spinach Salad Sautéed shrimp, peppers and mushrooms Balsamic Vinaigrette
Chicken Breast Broccoli Side salad	Salmon Roasted asparagus and bok choy

Day 3

16 oz. water
1 cup of hot lemon
water enhanced with
raw apple cider vinegar
and cayenne pepper
Green drink

Bulletproof style coffee
or tea (1 tablespoon
coconut oil and 1
tablespoon grass-fed
butter)

Massaged Kale Salad
Raw blue cheese, sun
flower seeds, dried
Cranberries
Turkey

Scallops
Sautéed spinach with
garlic and ginger
Sautéed pea pods with
maitake mushrooms

Day 4

16 oz. water
1 cup of hot lemon
water enhanced with
raw apple cider vinegar
and cayenne pepper
Green drink

Bulletproof style coffee
or tea (1 tablespoon
coconut oil and 1
tablespoon grass-fed
butter)

Mixed Greens Salad
Lump crab meat and
asparagus
Lime vinaigrette

Chicken Fajita on Sweet
Potato
Side salad

Day 5

16 oz. water
1 cup of hot lemon
water enhanced with
raw apple cider vinegar
and cayenne pepper
Green drink

Bulletproof style coffee
or tea (1 tablespoon
coconut oil and 1
tablespoon grass-fed
butter)

Winter Squash Soup
Side Salad

Grass-fed Filet Mignon
Arugula salad
Broccoli

Day 6

16 oz. water
1 cup of hot lemon
water enhanced with
raw apple cider vinegar
and cayenne pepper
Green drink

Bulletproof style coffee
or tea (1 tablespoon
coconut oil and 1
tablespoon grass-fed
butter)

Mixed Greens Salad
Salmon, red cabbage,
shredded carrot, roasted
corn, red bell pepper
Balsamic vinaigrette

Vegetable omelet
Side salad

Day 7

16 oz. water
1 cup of hot lemon
water enhanced with
raw apple cider vinegar
and cayenne pepper
Green drink

Bulletproof style coffee
or tea (1 tablespoon
coconut oil and 1
tablespoon grass-fed
butter)

Crudité and hummus
Olives and nuts

Turkey Bolognese
Spaghetti Squash
Caesar Salad

Shopping Guidelines

1. Buy organic. Since your goal is to decrease your toxic load and improve your body's health and vitality, you want to avoid traditionally farmed produce as they use pesticides. All pesticides kill bugs by poisoning their nervous systems, but those same chemicals directly affect your mitochondria, brain, nervous system, and the essential bacteria in your gut.

   Organic produce may cost slightly more than traditionally farmed produce, but the benefits far outweigh the cost. The bottom line is that you can pay now (buy organic) or you can pay later (disease and death), but you will pay.

2. Fresh is best. Many grocery stores are responding to the increased demand for fresh, organic produce options. Farmers markets are also a good source of local, fresh produce.

   If you live in an area that does not have an abundance of options for fresh, organic vegetables and fruit, then frozen produce is the next best option. Frozen produce is usually harvested at its peak and processed within a short time; thus, it retains more nutrients and enzymes than that of the canned variety.

3. Choose only clean meat, such as wild-caught, sustainable fish; organic, free-range poultry and eggs; pasture-raised pork; and grass-fed bison or beef. If you are committed to consuming dairy, opt for grass-fed, organic dairy products. Keeping it clean will help to reduce your exposure to added hormones, antibiotics, and other toxins.

4. Use olive oil and coconut oil to meet most of your cooking needs. Acceptable olive oil needs to be extra virgin, organic, and cold pressed. It is important to protect the oil because light affects the polyphenols, making the oil rancid and decreasing the health benefits. Avoid oil in clear containers; olive oil sold in a tin or crock is preferred. Always store oil in a cabinet, not on the counter. And while you may love some incredible Italian or Greek olive oil

(who doesn't?), imported oil tends to be much older than the oil produced in California.

5. Use honey if necessary. Limit sweetener to a *small* amount of honey, raw (unpasteurized). Don't overdo it!

6. Choose sea salt or pink Himalayan salt. They contain essential minerals.

7. The bulk food section has an abundance of economical options for nuts, seeds, and legumes. These are important sources of protein.

   Canned beans cost more than the dried version, but they are also very convenient. So if you do buy canned, choose organic in BPA-free cans.

8. Don't forget to stock up on mitochondrial superfoods:

   Meats: liver, lamb, sardines, anchovies, tuna, oysters, wild-caught Alaskan salmon

   Seeds and nuts: cashews, pumpkin seeds, almonds, walnuts

   Fruit and veggies: spinach, kale, Swiss chard, cabbage, broccoli, onions, garlic, avocado, banana, berries

Meal Prep

It takes some time to prepare fresh meals. In the beginning, deciding what you are going to eat and planning your meals for the week can be time-consuming. Hopefully these tips will make it easier and you will have fun experimenting in a whole new world of culinary adventures.

It is important to eat a variety of food. Your quest for health and an extended health span will be short-lived if you eat the same thing day in and day out. It will not be sustainable. Eat the rainbow and try new vegetables and new preparations. You may not like everything you try, but you may be surprised at the number of new things that you are excited to eat.

Case in point, my partner's boys were not frequent vegetable consumers. Over time I introduced a wide variety of options. Interestingly enough, their favorites are now broccoli, asparagus, bok choy, and salad in its many forms. As they tried new things, they opened up their minds and palates to the new tastes and textures. Kids *can* learn to love vegetables!

1. Make a list. This will save you time at the store and prevent you from making emotional purchases. There are many options for alkaline recipes. Peruse Pinterest and vegetarian food blogs for ideas—not because you need to become a vegetarian or vegan, but because they offer creative ways to prepare and enjoy vegetables—and look at Whole30 recipes.

2. Shop only one to two times per week. This will save you time and money. When you plan your meals for the week, you will know how much produce you will use, so just buy what you need, avoiding the need to throw away old, unused produce.

3. Keep it simple. Most meals can be prepared in thirty minutes or less. I save more complex and time-consuming recipes for the weekend when I have more time to invest.

4. Try to eat 50 percent of your alive food intake in its raw form. For the rest, lightly steam, quickly stir fry, or roast the vegetables. You will maintain the nutrients and enzymes by not overcooking.

5. Stage your meal plans. By this I mean think about chopping enough onions at one time to fulfill your upcoming meals, keep them in a glass container, and use them throughout the week. Same goes for meat. If you have a roast chicken early in the week, you can add leftovers to a salad for lunch or use them in a soup or stir fry later in the week.

6. Keep some snacks prepared and readily available. I always have crudité in my refrigerator. I clean and cut a mix of vegetables that can be enjoyed raw and keep them in a glass bowl filled with water. They are visible and accessible whenever anyone opens the refrigerator looking for "something to eat." Nuts and seeds are also great snack options.

Healing Crisis

I mentioned the healing crisis previously in the book, but I think it is important to revisit it again. All eight practices will have a detoxifying effect throughout your body, even practice 8: Gratitude. Unhealthy food and additive addictions and withdrawals can be a very real part of detoxification. In addition, your GI tract, as well as other parts of your body, has stored poisons and drugs enveloped in your fat cells. This compartmentalization is the body's will to survive under any conditions. During detoxification these time capsules can be broken down and the contents may temporarily flood the blood and tax the liver and kidneys. The detoxification process can have temporary annoying effects as the toxins are being eliminated. These symptoms include, but are not limited to disorientation, nausea, pain, headache, zingers, dizziness, etc. The process of detoxification can be subtle, and at times profound.

The important thing to remember is that the symptoms associated with the release of toxins, whether or not they are physical or emotional, are a normal part of the healing process. And while they may be temporarily uncomfortable, they will not persist. These are not reasons or rationalizations for you to withdraw from the program, they are an indication that you must continue so the toxic burden is lifted.

Liberating toxins is the one of the most important parts of any health restoration program, or weight loss program for that matter. One of the functions of the fat stores in our bodies is to bind and isolate toxins, such as mercury, heavy metals, pesticides, and chemicals. Whether or not they are swallowed, smoked, injected or absorbed, these toxins bio-accumulate in your fat, impacting your body as a whole. According to Walter Crinnion, an expert in Environmental Medicine, more than four hundred chemical contaminants have been found in human fat. No one is immune to this. For this reason, even a fairly healthy adult of normal weight who rarely gets sick can benefit from the practices in this book and their associated detoxification effects.

The metabolic systems and pathways of the body are intricate and diverse, but simply put: if there is no way to bind these toxins and escort them from the body through the colon and kidneys, the body will continue to produce and store fat to isolate the toxins in an effort of self-preservation. Many cases of weight loss resistance or the inability to keep weight off is caused by this phenomenon.

Here are some ways to help get you through this healing crisis with ease:
1. Drink water!
2. Eat lots of green, leafy vegetables.
3. Breathe.
4. Exercise every day.
5. Love yourself and be proud of your efforts.

Just don't stop! Better health, abundant energy, and a vibrant life await you on this journey.

Recipes

"Success is the sum of small efforts, repeated day in and day out."

—Robert Collier

It is important to eat enough food—you should not feel deprived or hungry—so during the transition into better eating, you may need to amp up your alive food intake. But your cravings will cease, I promise, usually within a couple weeks. Remember your brain will be looking for its dopamine fix, usually in the form of sugar. This can be a strong driver of behavior and a quick way to derail your success.

The following recipes focus on providing you with plenty of options to get your ten servings of vegetables. I have also included a few that contain meat or fish in the recipe, but for the most part, they are vegetable-centric.

Recipes often provide me with inspiration; however, I rarely measure everything out and follow them exactly. This habit really irritated my mom when she was trying to instill in me proper cooking and baking skills.

The upside of my creativity has been a plethora of outstanding meals. The downside is that I rarely create the same thing twice.

With that in mind, I have done my best to estimate the ingredient amounts. Again, I hope to inspire you with vegetables, and you can borrow my ideas until your own creativity takes hold. These recipes will give you some diversity to get you started.

You will notice that I have not included any traditional dietary equivalent information, such as proteins, carbohydrates, fats, sugar, or calories. I do not promote counting calories, the Standard American Diet, or the food pyramid. Instead I recommend that you give your body what it needs and eliminate what it doesn't. We all can benefit from eating more vegetables and monitoring your pH will help to guide you on how many you personally need to eat to optimize your health.

Remember, you do not have to become a vegetarian or vegan to achieve health. Alive vegetables should comprise 80 percent of your food intake on a daily basis. So, pull out your knives and apron and get chopping!

Dip It

Hummus

1 can garbanzo beans, drained, liquid reserved (or cook 1 cup dried beans in a slow cooker on high for 4 hours and add 4 cups of water and 1 teaspoon baking soda)

1 teaspoon salt

½ teaspoon pepper

1 teaspoon cumin

¼ – ½ teaspoon cayenne pepper

2–3 garlic cloves

⅓ cup tahini

Juice of 2 lemons

¼ cup Italian parsley

Place all ingredients into a food processor and pulse until smooth. Add reserved bean liquid a little at a time to achieve desired consistency. Adjust seasoning to taste.

Serve with assorted crudité.

Guacamole

3 ripe avocados

¾ cup cherry tomatoes, diced (I like the mini-plum variety for this)

1 jalapeño, minced

½ cup cilantro, coarsely chopped

2 tablespoons freshly squeezed lime juice

1–2 teaspoons of salt, to taste

Pepper

Cut each avocado in half and remove the pit. Slice into cubes inside the skin and then scoop into a medium-sized bowl. Add remaining ingredients, and then gently mash with a potato masher or fork, maintaining a relatively chunky texture.

Makes about 3 cups.

Serve with assorted crudité.

Pico de Gallo

6 Roma tomatoes, seeded and diced small

½ cup finely diced sweet onion

⅓ cup chopped fresh cilantro

1 jalapeño pepper, seeded and minced

2 tablespoons fresh lime juice

Salt

Makes 3 cups. This is best if used the same day. This simple sauce is great on salads, chicken, or fish.

Peak of the Season Pesto

2 ½ cups fresh basil, firmly packed

½ cup parmesan cheese, grated

2 garlic cloves

½ cup olive oil

½ cup pine nuts

Salt to taste

Combine all ingredients except for the olive oil in a blender or food processor. Blend until well mixed. Then add the olive oil in a slow, steady stream until a smooth texture is achieved.

Pesto goes beyond pasta. Add it to fish, chicken, or spaghetti squash. You can also add it as a garnish for soups.

This may be refrigerated for several weeks in a lidded jar. Add a thin layer of olive oil to prevent oxidation.

You can also freeze pesto in an ice cube tray for the perfect individual serving size portion. Transfer frozen cubes to a freezer safe bag or container. If you plan to freeze, however, you need to leave out the cheese.

Mango Salsa

3 Ataúlfo mangos, pitted, peeled, and diced

½ cup cilantro, minced

1 red bell pepper, diced

Juice of 1 lime

1 jalapeño pepper, diced

Salt

Combine all ingredients in a bowl and toss. Adjust seasoning to taste. This is a great topping for fish, chicken, or tacos.

Makes approximately 2 cups

Soups

Winter Squash Soup

1 medium butternut squash, halved lengthwise with seeds removed

1 kabocha squash, halved with seeds removed

1 medium sweet onion, diced

6 cups of vegetable or chicken broth

Extra virgin olive oil

Sea salt and pepper

Preheat oven to 375 degrees. Rub olive oil on flesh side of squash and place oiled-side down on a baking sheet. Add about ½" of water to sheet. Bake 1 hour or until squash is very soft and easily squeezed with tender pressure.

While squash is cooling slightly, sauté the onion in olive oil until it just starts to caramelize. Scoop 1 squash into blender, add half of the broth, and blend until smooth. Transfer to a soup pot. Add remaining squash, onions, remaining broth, sea salt, and pepper to blender, then process until smooth. Transfer to soup pot.

Gently simmer for 20 minutes. Add more broth (or water) if soup is too thick. Adjust seasoning to taste.

Serves 6

Topping options:

Diced roasted red pepper and roasted pumpkin seeds

Snipped chives and orange zest

Crispy Brussels sprouts

Crispy bacon or pancetta bits

Pesto

Cauliflower Curry Soup

1 sweet onion, diced

3 garlic cloves, minced

2 stalks of celery, diced

1 medium- to large-sized cauliflower, cored and cut into florets

1 teaspoon curry powder

1 teaspoon cumin

2 cups coconut milk, depending on desired consistency may need a little extra water

½ teaspoon cayenne pepper

Salt and pepper

Olive oil

Cilantro for garnish

In a soup pot, sauté onion and celery in olive oil until onions are translucent and not yet browning. Add the cauliflower florets and spices, cook until tender.

Puree with coconut milk in a blender. You may need to work in batches. Return the soup to the stove top. Adjust seasonings and use a little water to thin if necessary. Top with minced cilantro.

Serves 4–6

Tomato Soup

2 pounds Italian tomatoes, quartered lengthwise

1 red bell pepper, cut into 8 pieces

1 sweet onion, diced

3 garlic cloves, minced

1 quart jar home-canned tomatoes or 28-ounce can of whole organic tomatoes, including juice

1–2 cups of bone broth or water

1 teaspoon fresh thyme leaves

2 cups of basil

½ cup Italian parsley

¼ –½ teaspoon crushed red pepper, depending on taste

Olive oil

Salt and pepper

Pine Nuts for garnish

Preheat oven to 400 degrees.

Toss the fresh tomatoes and red pepper with olive oil, salt, and pepper. Roast on a sheet pan for approximately 45 minutes.

In a soup pot, sauté the onions and garlic in olive oil until the onions are translucent. Add the canned tomatoes, roasted tomatoes and red pepper, and herbs and spices.

Blend in batches, using the bone broth (or water) to achieve your desired consistency. Return to soup pot and simmer for 30 to 40 minutes. Adjust seasoning to taste.

Delicious served hot or cold.

Serves 4–6

Delicata Squash and Spinach Soup

2 Delicata squash, peeled, seeded, and cubed

1 sweet onion, diced

3 garlic cloves, minced

6 cups of spinach

½ cup Italian parsley, minced

4 cups bone broth

2–4 cups water

1 teaspoon fresh thyme leaves

Olive oil

Salt and pepper

In a soup pot, sauté the onion and garlic in olive oil until the onions are translucent. Add squash and thyme. Season with about 1 teaspoon salt and ½ teaspoon black pepper. Continue to cook for about 5 minutes.

Add liquids, starting with 2 cups of water, and bring to a boil. Turn down to a simmer, add spinach and parsley. Simmer for 30 minutes or until squash is fork tender, adding additional water, if necessary, for broth volume. Adjust seasonings to taste.

Serves 4–6

Butternut Squash and Pear Soup

1 medium butternut squash, cleaned and cubed

1 large yam, peeled and cubed

1 large sweet onion, diced

3 pears, cored and cubed

2 cups bone broth

1 ½ cups water

⅓ cup dry white wine

¼ cup coconut milk

1 cinnamon stick

Fresh chives

2 tablespoons grass-fed butter

Salt and pepper

Combine the squash, yam, bone broth, water, cinnamon stick, and about 1 teaspoon of salt in a soup pot. Simmer until tender, about 40–45 minutes. Discard the cinnamon stick.

Sauté the onions in butter until they are translucent. Add the pears and continue cooking for another 5 minutes, stirring often to prevent the onions from browning too much. Add wine and simmer for another 10 minutes.

Puree in batches in a blender, adding coconut milk. Return to soup pot, adjust seasoning with salt and pepper. Then heat, but do not boil.

Garnish with snipped chives.

Serves 6

Bone Broth

2 pounds beef femur bones

1 pound ox tails

1 onion

1 fennel bulb

3 carrots

4 garlic cloves

4 celery stalks

Bunch Italian parsley

Fresh thyme

Fresh rosemary

Bay leaf

Pepper corns

Salt

2 tablespoons raw apple cider vinegar

Olive oil

Drizzle olive oil over bones and roast in oven at 400 degrees for 30 minutes. Add everything to a slow cooker and cover with water. Run two 10-hour cooking cycles. Strain out solids.

Enjoy a warm cup of bone broth periodically to help support your gut health. Add to soups in place of stock. Store in an airtight container in the refrigerator.

As an alternative you can use leftover poultry carcasses, generally 2 chicken or 1 turkey.

Dressings

Balsamic Dressing

½ cup good balsamic
vinegar

1 cup olive oil

1 tablespoon Dijon mustard

Place all ingredients in a jar with a lid and shake to combine.

Curry Dressing

2 garlic cloves

1 tablespoon honey

Zest of 1 orange

1 teaspoon cinnamon

1 teaspoon curry powder

Pinch of salt

½ cup seasoned rice vinegar

1 cup olive oil

In a blender or food processor, blend everything except for the olive oil for about 1 minute. Continue to blend while adding the oil in a slow continuous stream. The dressing will thicken nicely.

In addition to dressing the Quinoa Salad, I also like to use this dressing on a mixed green salad topped with roast chicken and toasted, chopped almonds. A little chèvre adds some decadence.

Tahini Garlic Dressing

½ cup tahini, preferably freshly ground

1 garlic clove, minced

¼ cup fresh lemon juice

½ cup water

2 tablespoons olive oil

2 teaspoons tamari

1 teaspoon raw apple cider vinegar

Generous pinch of black pepper

Blend all ingredients thoroughly in a blender or food processor. Keeps long-term if refrigerated.

This dressing is a great change of pace for a simple salad, especially as a side for lamb.

Lime Vinaigrette

6 tablespoons olive oil

3 tablespoons fresh lime juice

Zest of 2 limes

4 teaspoons rice wine vinegar

2 teaspoons freshly grated ginger

1 teaspoon honey

Salt and pepper

Place all ingredients in a lidded jar and shake to combine. Adjust seasoning to taste.

Mustard Vinaigrette

½ cup olive oil

2 tablespoons red wine vinegar

1 tablespoon freshly squeezed lemon juice

1 tablespoon Dijon mustard

1 garlic clove, pressed

Salt and pepper

Place all ingredients in a lidded jar and shake to combine. Adjust seasoning to taste.

Caesar Dressing

1 egg yolk

1 tablespoon Dijon mustard

2 tablespoons balsamic vinegar

2 garlic cloves

6 anchovy filets or 1 tablespoon anchovy paste

1 cup olive oil

Salt and pepper

Process all ingredients in a blender or food processor until smooth. While continuing to blend, add the olive oil in a thin stream. If the blender locks up due to the thickness of the dressing, add a tablespoon of warm water. You want to make sure to add all the olive oil. Adjust seasoning to taste.

This recipe makes enough for multiple salads and will keep in the refrigerator for a week or so. It is also delicious as a dip for steamed artichokes.

Makes 1 ½ cups

Salads

Quinoa Salad

3 cups cooked quinoa

1 cup finely chopped scallions, both white and green parts

1 carrot, shredded

2 stalks celery, diced

½ red pepper, diced

½ cup frozen peas

½ cup broccoli, blanched and diced

1 cup dried currants, cranberries or cherries

1 cup fresh Italian parsley, minced

½ teaspoon salt

½ cup seasoned rice vinegar (you may need to add a bit more if the salad is prepared in advance)

1 ½ cups Curry Dressing

Toss everything together in a medium-sized bowl and serve.

Serves 6

Arugula Salad

2 bundles of arugula, roughly chopped

½ small radicchio, sliced thin

1 handful watercress

½ red bell pepper, julienned

½ cup walnut pieces

4 ounces of Point Reyes blue cheese, sliced

Salt and pepper

1 persimmon, quartered and sliced thin cross-wise (peach, nectarine, or mango are good substitutes if persimmon is not available)

Wash and dry greens. Toss all ingredients in a salad bowl with balsamic dressing, salt, and pepper to taste and serve immediately.

Serves 4

Fresh Crab Salad

2 heads Bibb Lettuce or ½ pound romaine hearts

1 pound asparagus, tough ends removed

2 avocado, diced

1 pound fresh crab meat

Lime Vinaigrette

Steam asparagus until just tender. Place spears in an ice bath. Once cool toss with a ⅓ of the vinaigrette. Tear lettuce into bite-sized pieces, toss with a ⅓ of the vinaigrette and arrange on 4 plates. Toss crab with remaining vinaigrette. Divide among the 4 plates. Add avocado and asparagus to each plate and serve.

Serves 4

Chop Salad

1 head romaine, washed thoroughly and tough outer leaves removed

1 cup fresh basil leaves, cut into thin strips

1 ½ cups snap peas, strings removed and cut in half on the diagonal

2 ears of corn

2 cups garbanzo beans

1 cucumber, peeled, seeded, and diced

1 carrot, shredded

4 scallions, thinly sliced

½ red bell pepper, diced

½ cup radishes, sliced

½ cup artichoke hearts, chopped

1 cup cherry tomatoes, steamed and cut in half

½ cup Point Reyes blue cheese, crumbled

Mustard Vinaigrette

Blanch peas for 2 minutes and place in an ice bath. Blanch corn for 2 minutes and place in an ice bath. Cut romaine into thin strips and add to large salad bowl. Cut corn kernels from cobs and add to bowl. Add remaining ingredients and toss.

Serves 4

Niçoise Salad

8 ounces mixed spring greens

2 hard-boiled eggs, peeled and cut into eighths

8 ounces yellow fin tuna, seared for 3 minutes each side (or 1 can line-caught tuna packed in water without additives, drained)

1 cup green beans, lightly steamed

1 cup new potatoes, steamed and halved

1 cup cherry tomatoes, steamed and halved

½ cup olives

Arrange greens on a serving platter. Top with the remaining ingredients by arranging each ingredient in a row. Drizzle with balsamic dressing. Salt and pepper to taste.

Serves 2

Cabbage Slaw

½ head green cabbage (approximately 1 pound), cored and thinly sliced

½ head red cabbage (approximately ½ pound), cored and thinly sliced

4 large carrots, shredded

1 bunch Italian kale, ribs removed and thinly sliced

Toss all ingredients in a large bowl and top with dressing. Keep refrigerated.

Serves 6–8

Dressing

2 egg yolks

4 tablespoons diced onions

4 tablespoons raw apple cider vinegar

2 tablespoons honey

1 cup olive oil

Salt and pepper

In a food processor or blender, combine all ingredients except olive oil. Continue to blend and add the oil in a steady stream until the dressing thickens. Adjust seasoning to taste.

Kenna's Favorite Caesar

2 heads of romaine, washed, dried, and torn into bite-sized pieces

¾ cup shredded parmesan cheese

2 roasted chicken breasts, sliced

Caesar dressing

Add all ingredients to a large salad bowl. Toss with just enough dressing to lightly coat lettuce. Salmon makes a delicious alternative to chicken.

Serves 2

Spinach, Chicken and Pea Salad

8 ounces baby spinach

10 ounces frozen peas

2 roasted chicken breasts, cubed

½ cup pesto

½ cup grated parmesan cheese

4 tablespoons pine nuts

Salt and pepper

Wash and dry spinach. Put peas into a strainer and run under cold water to defrost. Place spinach, peas, and chicken into a large salad bowl. Add the pesto and cheese, then toss to combine ingredients. Divide among 4 plates. Top each with 1 tablespoon of pine nuts. Season to taste with salt and pepper.

Serves 4

Butternut Squash Salad

1 medium butternut squash, peeled, seeded, and diced into 1-inch pieces

½ sweet onion, sliced into half rounds

8 ounces mixed greens

½ cup walnuts

4 ounces chèvre, crumbled

Olive oil

Salt and pepper

Balsamic dressing

Preheat oven to 400 degrees.

Place squash and onion slices on a sheet pan and drizzle with olive oil. Toss and add salt and pepper. Roast for 20 minutes, turning once.

Place mixed greens in a large salad bowl. Add the roasted vegetables, walnuts, and chèvre. Use just enough dressing to moisten the greens. Toss well and serve immediately.

Serves 4

Best Fresh Herb Caprese Salad

8 ounces mixed greens

2 ripe heirloom tomatoes, sliced

8 ounces fresh buffalo mozzarella

2 teaspoons fresh thyme

2 teaspoons fresh oregano, chopped

12 fresh basil leaves, thinly sliced

Pesto

Balsamic vinegar

Salt and pepper

Arrange greens on a serving platter. Layer the tomato slices to cover and distribute mozzarella chunks. Sprinkle herbs. Drizzle pesto and balsamic vinegar. Generously salt and pepper.

Serves 4

Plenty of Green Salad

1 cup baby chard or spinach

1 cup baby kale

½ pound haricot verts

2 cups snow peas

10 ounces frozen peas, thawed

¼ cup red onion, finely chopped

Zest of 1 lemon

2 tablespoons tarragon, chopped

1 tablespoon sesame seeds

Salt and pepper

Mustard Vinaigrette

Bring a medium saucepan of water to a boil. Blanch the green beans for 4 minutes and then transfer to an ice bath. Blanch the snow peas for 1 minute and transfer to an ice bath. Dry the vegetables.

In a large salad bowl, combine chard, kale, green beans, snow peas, peas, and onion. Dress with mustard vinaigrette. Add the zest, tarragon, and sesame seeds. Season to taste with salt and pepper. Toss once more and serve.

Serves 4

Terri's Holiday Salad

1 pound of mixed greens

4 clementines, peeled and separated into sections

⅓ cup walnuts, chopped

½ cup pomegranate arils

⅓ cup fig balsamic vinegar

¼ cup olive oil

Whisk the vinegar and oil together in the bottom of a large salad bowl. Add salt and pepper to taste, then add remaining ingredients. Toss just before serving.

Serves 6–8

Sprout Slaw

1 pound of Brussels sprouts, trimmed and shredded

1 bunch Italian kale, stems removed and thinly sliced

1 green apple, cored and diced

4 scallions, white and green parts thinly sliced

1 cucumber, peeled and seeded, diced

½ cup walnuts, chopped

Handful of dried cranberries

Salt and pepper

Mustard vinaigrette

Combine all ingredients, except vinaigrette, in a large salad bowl. Toss to combine. Dress with vinaigrette to coat shredded leaves. Let sit for 5 minutes. Toss again, season to taste, and add additional vinaigrette if too dry.

Serves 4

Massaged Kale Salad

8 ounces baby kale

½ lemon

Point Reyes blue cheese, crumbled

Sunflower seeds

Dried cranberries

Salt and pepper

Generously salt kale in a large salad bowl. Add lemon juice, a drizzle of olive oil, and some fresh cracked pepper. Toss for 2–3 minutes until the leaves start to wilt slightly. Adjust seasoning to taste. Plate the greens and top with cheese, sunflower seeds, and cranberries.

Experiment with toppings to keep things interesting.

Serves 4

Taco Salad

1 pound of ground turkey or bison

1 sweet onion, diced

2 garlic gloves, minced

½ red bell pepper, diced

½ green bell pepper, diced

1 jalapeño pepper, minced

1 bunch cilantro, minced

1 teaspoon cumin

1 teaspoon coriander

1 tablespoon chili powder

¼ teaspoon cayenne

Olive oil

Salt and pepper

Avocado, diced

2 radishes, sliced

Pico de gallo or mango salsa

8 ounces mixed greens or Bibb lettuce to do wraps

Sauté onion, garlic, and peppers in olive oil over medium-high heat until onions are translucent. Add ground meat and continue to cook until browned. Add spices and stir to thoroughly combine; season with salt and pepper.

Top lettuce with meat and garnish with avocado, radish, and salsa of your choice.

Serves 4–6

Vegetables

Sautéed Spinach with Garlic and Ginger

3 garlic cloves, minced

1 tablespoon fresh grated ginger

2 tablespoons tamari

¼ cup sesame seeds

1 ½ tablespoons olive oil

2 teaspoons toasted sesame oil

10–12 cups fresh spinach (you can also use beet greens, Swiss chard or kale, or a combination)

In a large skillet add oils and warm over medium-high heat. Add the garlic and ginger and sauté until just starting to turn brown, roughly 2–3 minutes. Add spinach and continue to cook another 2–3 minutes. Add the tamari and sesame seeds. Salt and pepper to taste.

Serves 4

*If serving with seared scallops, just wipe out the skillet with a paper towel. Add olive oil and sesame oil in same amounts as above and heat over medium-high flame. Dry 2 pounds of fresh sea scallops with a paper towel and salt and pepper to taste. Sear scallops until dark golden brown.

Butternut Squash Gratin

1 medium butternut squash, peeled and cubed

3 garlic cloves, minced

2 leeks, halved and sliced (approximately 2 cups)

1 red bell pepper, diced

3 cups wild mushrooms, sliced

4 tomatoes, sliced

¼ cup fresh Italian parsley, minced

¼ cup fresh herbs, minced (I like fresh basil, thyme, and oregano)

¾ cup walnuts, chopped

1 cup parmesan, grated

Olive oil

Salt and pepper

Toss squash with some olive oil and salt and pepper. Bake on a cookie sheet at 375 degrees for 30 minutes, until easily pierced with a fork.

Sauté garlic, leeks, and red pepper in olive oil for 5 minutes over medium heat. Transfer to a bowl.

Sauté the mushrooms in olive oil over medium heat until lightly browned. Lightly salt.

Lightly oil an 8x11 baking dish. Layer the ingredients in the following order: squash, mushrooms, the garlic veggie mixture, tomatoes, salt and pepper, herbs, walnuts, and cheese. Bake at 350 degrees covered for 30 minutes and uncovered for another 10 minutes to brown the top.

It goes beautifully with a mixed green salad or roast chicken.

Serves 4

Yvonne's Chard

3 bunches chard (about 12 cups of cleaned loosely packed leaves)

2 garlic cloves, minced

1 lemon, halved

¼ teaspoon red pepper flakes

¼ cup olive oil

Salt and pepper

Stem and wash chard well. Dry leaves. Slice into 1-inch strips. Heat a large sauté pan with the oil and red pepper flakes over a medium-high flame. Add the chard and garlic. Stir occasionally. When the leaves are wilted, season to taste with salt and pepper and squeeze in the lemon, being careful to catch the seeds. Serve immediately.

Serves 4

Steamed Artichokes

4 large artichokes

1 lemon, sliced

2 tablespoons balsamic vinegar

Caesar dressing or tahini garlic dressing

Trim the artichoke stems so they sit flat. Slice off the top inch or so of each artichoke. Place artichokes stem side down in a stockpot that is large enough for them to sit side by side without crowding. Drizzle balsamic dressing over them. Add 2 inches of water and the lemon slices. Cover and bring to a boil; lower heat and simmer for 45 minutes to an hour. Artichokes are done when a knife can easily pierce through the base. Drain. Serve with a side of Caesar dressing for dipping.

Serves 4

Brussels Sprout Sauté

1 pound of Brussels sprouts, trimmed and sliced

½ sweet onion, diced

1 clove garlic, minced

¼ teaspoon crushed red pepper flakes

1 tablespoon grass-fed butter

Olive oil

1 tablespoon thick, syrupy and sweet Balsamic vinegar

Salt and pepper

Sauté Brussels sprouts, onion, garlic, and crushed red pepper flakes in olive oil over medium-high flame for 5–7 minutes. Brussels sprouts should be crisp and tender. Add butter, salt, and pepper. Drizzle with balsamic vinegar.

Serves 4

Crispy Brussels Sprouts

10 Brussels sprouts, sliced

8 shiitake mushroom caps, thinly sliced

¼ cup hazelnuts, loosely chopped

1 tablespoon fresh sage, finely chopped

Balsamic vinegar

Extra virgin olive oil

Salt and pepper

Preheat the oven to 400 degrees. Combine all ingredients on a baking sheet or pan, toss with olive oil, balsamic vinegar, salt, and pepper. Bake for 10–15 minutes, stirring occasionally to avoid burning. When slightly crispy, remove from oven and serve hot.

Serves 2

Roasted Brussels Sprouts

1 pound of Brussels sprouts, trimmed and cut in half through core

4 ounces pancetta, diced

1 tablespoon thick, syrupy and sweet balsamic vinegar

Orange zest

Olive oil

Salt and pepper

Preheat oven to 400 degrees.

Place Brussels sprouts and pancetta on a sheet pan and drizzle with olive oil. Toss well and distribute into a single layer. Season generously with salt and pepper. Roast for 20–30 minutes, turn once during roasting. Remove from oven and drizzle with balsamic vinegar. Sprinkle with orange zest and adjust seasoning to taste.

Serves 4

Roasted Broccolini

1 bunch broccolini

Olive oil

Salt and pepper

Lemon zest

Preheat oven to 375 degrees.

Trim the tough ends off broccolini. Place in a single layer on a sheet pan. Overcrowding will cause them to steam rather than roast. Drizzle with olive oil and toss. Season with salt and pepper. Roast for 15 minutes until the stems are crisp and tender. Sprinkle with lemon zest and serve.

Serves 1

Roasted Cauliflower

1 large head of cauliflower, cored and sliced into ¾ inch slices

8 ounces mushrooms, sliced

½ sweet onion, diced

1 garlic clove, minced

Shredded parmesan cheese

6–8 peppadew peppers, diced

2 scallions, white and green parts minced

4 tablespoons pine nuts

Olive oil

Salt and pepper

Preheat oven to 375 degrees.

Place cauliflower steaks on a sheet pan. Drizzle with olive oil and season generously with salt and pepper. Make sure to address both sides. Bake for 30 minutes, turning once. Cauliflower should be tender and just starting to brown.

While cauliflower is roasting, sauté onion, mushrooms, and garlic in olive oil over medium heat until tender and caramelized. Season with salt and pepper.

Top the roasted cauliflower with mushroom mixture. Sprinkle with cheese and return to the oven for an additional 2 minutes. Distribute the diced peppers, scallions, and pine nuts evenly.

Serves 4–6

Mashed Cauliflower

1 head cauliflower, cored
and broken into pieces

3 tablespoons grass-fed
butter

Coconut milk

Salt and pepper

Steam the cauliflower until tender. Puree cauliflower in a food processor with butter. Slowly drizzle coconut milk until a creamy texture is attained. Season with salt and pepper to taste.

This is a great accompaniment to most meat and fish.

Serves 4

Roasted Beets

6 small- to medium-sized
assorted beets (red, golden,
Chioggia)

Handful of microgreens

Feta or chèvre, optional

Balsamic vinegar

Salt and pepper

Preheat oven to 375 degrees.

Remove stems, leaving about ½ inch. Scrub beets and wrap each beet in parchment paper and then aluminum foil. Roast in oven for about 1 hour or until the beets "give" with a gentle squeeze. They should be firm, but not hard.

Remove wrappers and cut off the top and stem. The skin will easily separate and peel off by applying pressure with your thumb. Cut into cubes. If using multi-colored beets, keep each in a separate container until just prior to serving to avoid the red beets bleeding on to the yellow ones. Drizzle with balsamic and season to taste with salt and pepper. Combine beets and serve topped with microgreens and crumbled feta or chèvre if you desire.

Serves 2

Some Protein

Lime Marinated Salmon

⅓ cup freshly squeezed lime juice

1 sweet onion, diced

3 garlic cloves, minced

2 jalapeños, minced

1 bunch cilantro, coarsely chopped

1 tablespoon honey

¼ cup olive oil

1 teaspoon salt

2 pounds salmon

Combine marinade ingredients in a blender or food processor, pulse for 30 seconds. Pour half of the marinade over the bottom of a glass baking dish. Place fish on the marinade and pour the remaining marinade to cover the fish.

Marinade for at least 1 hour. Wipe excess marinade from the salmon, sprinkle with salt and pepper, grill or roast to desired doneness.

Serves 6–8

One Sheet Salmon Supper

2 pounds salmon

Olive oil

1 pound of asparagus

Salt and pepper

6 baby bok choy

Fennel salt

Trim tough ends off the asparagus. Cut the bok choy in half the long way. Toss vegetables with olive oil, salt, and pepper. Place the vegetables on ⅔ of a sheet pan. Place the salmon on the remaining ⅓ of the sheet pan. Sprinkle with fennel salt and pepper.

Roast in a 400-degree oven for approximately 20 minutes or until desired doneness.

Serves 6

Turkey Bolognese
with Spaghetti Sauce

1 large or 2 small spaghetti squash

1 sweet onion, diced

3 garlic cloves, minced

1 large carrot, shredded

1 celery stalk, diced

1 green bell pepper, diced

½ pound crimini mushrooms, sliced

2 cups spinach, sliced

1 pound of ground, organic turkey

1 quart of home-canned tomatoes or 28-ounce can of whole organic tomatoes, including juice or 3 pounds fresh Italian tomatoes, roasted

½ cup basil, thinly sliced

½ cup Italian parsley, chopped

½ teaspoon crushed red pepper

Olive oil

Salt and pepper

Preheat oven to 350 degrees.

Split spaghetti squash lengthwise and scrape out seeds with a spoon and discard. Place the squash cut side down on a rimmed baking sheet. Add ¼ inch of water to the sheet.

Bake squash until it is easily pierced with a fork, about 45 minutes. Remove from oven and scrape the squash strands into a colander.

Prepare the sauce while the squash is baking. In a large skillet, sauté onion and garlic in olive oil until translucent. Add carrot, celery, green pepper, and mushrooms. Continue cooking until mushrooms are glossy, but firm. Add turkey, crushed red pepper, salt, and pepper. Continue cooking until the turkey is browned.

Add tomatoes, basil, parsley, and spinach. Let sauce simmer and reduce for about 20–30 minutes. Add a splash of red wine if too much liquid has evaporated.

Top squash with sauce. Top with grated raw parmesan cheese.

Serves 6

Chicken Fajitas

2 organic boneless, skinless chicken breasts sliced into thin strips

½ sweet onion, diced

½ green bell pepper, sliced into strips

½ red bell pepper, sliced into strips

1 jalapeño, diced

1 cup sliced crimini mushrooms

1 teaspoon cumin

½ teaspoon coriander

½ teaspoon smoked paprika

Olive oil

Salt and pepper

½ cup chopped cilantro

½ lime

1 avocado, diced

2 sweet potatoes

Preheat oven to 350 degrees. Poke sweet potatoes several times with a knife and bake until they give with gentle pressure when squeezed, approximately 45 minutes.

In a large skillet sauté the onion and peppers in olive oil over medium-high heat until onions just start to become translucent. Add mushrooms, chicken, cumin, coriander, salt, and pepper. Continue cooking until the chicken is cooked through. Add paprika.

Slice cooked sweet potatoes into halves, lengthwise. Place halves cut side up on a serving platter. Top with chicken mixture. Add avocado, then squeeze lime over each potato and garnish with cilantro.

Serves 4

Eggs Benedict(less)

1 tomato, sliced

1 avocado, halved, pitted, peeled, and sliced

Handful of fresh baby spinach

2 poached eggs

1 teaspoon fresh, snipped chives

Splash of picante if you must

Using a slice of tomato as the base, top with avocado slices, spinach leaves, and a poached egg. Finish with chives, salt, pepper, and optional picante.

Serves 2

French Omelet

3 eggs

4 spears of asparagus, steamed

Chèvre, broken into marble-size pieces

Salt and pepper

Tarragon

Using a wire whisk, beat eggs until frothy and light. Salt and pepper to taste. Cook eggs over medium heat in a non-stick skillet. When the eggs are almost cooked through, add the asparagus to one half and cover the entire surface with chèvre pieces. Turn off heat and cover for 1 minute. Fold the omelet in half. Garnish with chopped tarragon.

Serves 2

Endless Option Scramble

2 eggs

1 cup vegetables

2 tablespoons fresh herbs

½ tomato, diced

½ avocado, diced

1 tablespoon grass-fed butter

Salt and pepper

Sauté vegetables in butter over medium heat until tender. Whisk eggs in a small bowl until light and frothy. Add eggs to vegetables, stirring occasionally until eggs are cooked through. Add herbs, mix, and serve.

Serves 1

Example combinations:

Onion, mushroom, spinach, Italian parsley, thyme

Onion, red bell pepper, wild mushroom, cilantro, chives

Leftover Yvonne's chard

Broccoli, basil, and chives

Asparagus, roasted red pepper, chanterelle mushrooms, thyme, chives, Italian parsley

Best Roast Chicken

1 whole, organic chicken

1 can cheap beer

Cayenne

Salt and pepper

Wash and dry chicken. Generously season with salt and pepper. Dust lightly with cayenne. Empty ⅓ of the beer and then perch the chicken on the beer can by inserting the can into the chicken's butt. Place in a baking dish. Roast at 375 degrees for 1 hour. Skin will be crispy and juices will run clear. Carve and serve.

Seared Tuna

2 pounds sashimi-grade fresh tuna steak

2 avocados, diced

¼ red onion, thinly sliced into half rounds

8 ounces mixed greens

2 scallions, white and green parts minced

2 tablespoons sesame seeds

3 freshly squeezed limes

Lime zest from 2 limes

1 teaspoon wasabi, either powder or prepared paste

2 teaspoons of tamari

1 teaspoon toasted sesame oil

Brush olive oil onto each side of the tuna steak. Allow skillet to preheat over high flame. Sauté fish for 2–3 minutes per side. Fish will be seared on the outside and raw in the center. Cool slightly before cutting into bite-sized cubes. Combine tuna, avocado, and onion in a bowl. To a lidded jar, add ¼ cup olive oil, lime juice, lime zest, wasabi, tamari, and sesame oil. Shake to combine. Add to bowl with tuna and toss gently. Divide greens onto 4 plates. Top with tuna–avocado mixture. Sprinkle scallions and sesame seeds on each salad portion.

Serves 4

Acknowledgements

I have been blessed with many incredible mentors and influencers throughout my life. They have all helped me to learn the lessons of life and business, and most importantly to find my voice.

My family provided me with an environment that encouraged learning and seeing possibilities even when they were not obvious. They instilled in me a positive value system and a strong work ethic. Without their leadership I would not be who I am today.

The honor of raising two beautiful daughters has inspired me to lead and guide with patience and compassion. I am humbled by their unwavering confidence and belief in my abilities as a woman, mother, doctor and entrepreneur.

My partner remained open-minded and supportive throughout the entire book writing process from concept to print. He patiently listened without judgement and embraced my rollercoaster of emotions. I am confident that he is as happy as I am that the book is finally finished (now we will actually be able to eat at the dining room table).

My tribe, especially the Dirty Girls, has encouraged me and lifted me up. It has been a long, strange trip and they have been there at my side going the distance with me. Their willingness to be research subjects in my cleanses, eating strategies and recipe development goes beyond the bounds of friendship. They elevate my spirit and bring joy to my life.

My dear friend Kate Dixon is an incredible project manager and designer. She not only helped to keep me focused and on schedule, she also transformed my words and vision to create the images contained within the book. She is a true rock star!

Lauren Reisfeld brought joy and laughter to the task of photos. She confidently directed the photo shoot and infused her ideas. She truly captured the essence of my vision.

Self-Publishing School was instrumental in making the process of writing this book actually do-able. Chandler Bolt and Scott Allen kept me inspired and motivated to finish this book. Their encouragement was abundant.

Katie Chambers with Beacon Pointe Services helped to refine my book with her edits. She was insightful and inquisitive, which forced me to build a stronger message. She helped to bring out the best in me and this book.

Tracy Atkins with The Book Makers really brought this book to the finish line. He swooped in like an angel and took the weight of the world off my shoulders. His experience, confidence and insight transformed my basic manuscript into this work of art.

Next Steps

8 Daily Practices 21-day Challenge

One of the biggest obstacles for most health seekers in implementing the practices contained within this book is that they don't have the right strategy or focus to begin with.

They don't know what to expect or where to start. A major life overhaul seems daunting. So instead of moving forward, they file it away for a later date when it might be more convenient.

That's why I want to provide you with a clear action plan on what to do next. How to take what you've just learned and put it into practice.

We'll start by dividing a 21-day time frame into three 7-day phases.

Each phase will focus on a radical gradualism approach to creating your own daily ritual incorporating the 8 Daily Practices.

It'll help you remove the roadblocks so you can stick to a plan and put it into place. It will also allow you to identify where your gaps are and get started on filling those in.

But most of it all, it will allow you to create a plan for establishing sustainable life habits that will optimize your health and healing potential. Building the foundation so that you can thrive.

And if you're ready to dive into creating consistent, predictable results, join the FREE 21-day Challenge where I guide you step-by-step in creating your own personalized health strategy!

You can learn more here:
www.drnancymiggins.com/21-day-challenge

DAYS 1-7: PHASE ONE

Over the next 7 days, you're going to focus identifying your starting point and your first destination on your journey. The goal is to be conscious, objective and accepting of the reality of your current state of health and well-being.

DAYS 8-14: PHASE TWO

In this next 7-day phase, you will focus increasing positive lifestyle behaviors. No shame or judgement about where you are, only grace and inspiration for where you want to be.

DAYS 15-21: PHASE THREE

In the last 7-days, you will focus on reducing and eliminating those lifestyle choices and behaviors that have negative consequences on your health and health potential. These things sabotage your efforts and impair your chance of success, both short-term and in the long run.

Get access to the 21-day Challenge at
www.drnancymiggins.com/21-day-challenge

Don't Go It Alone

If you are serious about making changes in your life and health, you need a support system. There is something magical that happens when you are accountable to someone else for following through with your commitments.

It is a win-win situation. Both you and your accountability buddy, or group, benefit from the support and encouragement. You help each other through the lows and celebrate the milestones. You are not alone!

Reach out to friends and family right now and ask them to join you during the 21-day Challenge. The quickest way to get them up to speed is to send them the link to www.drnancymiggins.com/8-practices-jumpstart so they can get free and immediate access to the **8 Daily Practices Jump Start Course**:

- Two FREE chapters of *Mastering the Health Continuum* book

- The FREE Introduction to the 8 Daily Practices video

- The FREE Introduction to the 8 Daily Practices audio

It will cost them nothing and you will be teaming up with someone who is also committed to taking control of their health and taking their quality of life to the next level. You can support, encourage and hold each other accountable.

IMPORTANT: Don't wait until you have an accountability partner to start the 8 Daily Practices 21-day Challenge. Whether or not you have found someone to embark on this journey with you, don't procrastinate. Start today, don't lose the inspiration, motivation and confidence that you have gained through reading this book.

Take action now. Get started. Then as soon as you can, invite a friend, family-member or co-worker to visit www.drnancymiggins.com/8-practices-jumpstart to get their FREE **8 Daily Practices Jump Start Course.**

In less than an hour they will be fully capable of being your 8 Daily Practices accountability partner. And, it is likely they will join you readily inspired!

Can You Help?

Thank You For Reading My Book!

I really appreciate all of your feedback, and I love hearing what you have to say.

I need your input to make the next version of this book and my future books better.

Please leave me an honest review on Amazon letting me know what you thought of the book.

Thanks so much!

Dr Nancy

Notes

Part 1

Romani M, Pistillo MP, Banelli B. Environmental epigenetics: crossroad between public health, lifestyle, and cancer prevention. *Biomed Res Int.* 2015;2015:587983. doi:10.1155/2015/587983

Pickles S[1], Vigié P[2], Youle RJ[3]. Mitophagy and quality control mechanisms in mitochondrial maintenance. *Curr Biol.* 2018;28(4):R170-R185. Published 2018 Feb 19. doi:10.1016/j.cub.2018.01.004

Jacomin AC, Taillebourg E, Fauvarque MO. Deubiquitinating enzymes related to autophagy: new therapeutic opportunities?. *Cells.* 2018;7(8):112. Published 2018 Aug 19. doi:10.3390/cells7080112

Martinez-Vicente M[1]. Neuronal mitophagy in neurodegenerative diseases. *Front Mol Neurosci.* 2017;10:64. Published 2017 Mar 8. doi:10.3389/fnmol.2017.00064. eCollection 2017.

Fivenson EM, Lautrup S, Sun N, et al. Mitophagy in neurodegeneration and aging. *Neurochem Int.* 2017;109:202–209. doi:10.1016/j.neuint.2017.02.007

Alirezaei M, Kemball CC, Flynn CT, Wood MR, Whitton JL, Kiosses WB. Short-term fasting induces profound neuronal autophagy. *Autophagy.* 2010;6(6):702–710. doi:10.4161/auto.6.6.12376

Patterson RE, Laughlin GA, LaCroix AZ, et al. Intermittent fasting and human metabolic health. *J Acad Nutr Diet.* 2015;115(8):1203–1212. doi:10.1016/j.jand.2015.02.018

Cline S. Mitochondrial DNA damage and its consequences for mitochondrial gene expression. *Biochim Biophys Acta.* 2012;1819(9-10):979-991. Published online 2012 Jun 19. doi:10.1016/j.bbagrm.2012.06.002

Salleh MR. Life event, stress and illness. *Malays J Med Sci.* 2008;15(4):9–18.

LaMattina, John. "The Biopharmaceutical Industry Provides 75% Of The FDA's Drug Review Budget. Is This A Problem?" Forbes.com.

https://www.forbes.com/sites/johnlamattina/2018/06/28/the-biopharmaceutical-industry-provides-75-of-the-fdas-drug-review-budget-is-this-a-problem/#22573a3749ec

World Health Organization. "Human Genomics in Global Health: Genes and noncommuniable diseases." Who.int.

https://www.who.int/genomics/public/geneticdiseases/en/index3.html

Thunders M. Epigenetics: its understanding is crucial to a sustainable healthcare system. *Healthcare (Basel).* 2015;3(2):194–204. Published 2015 Apr 1. doi:10.3390/healthcare3020194

Institute of Medicine (US) Committee on Assessing Interactions Among Social, Behavioral, and Genetic Factors in Health; Hernandez LM, Blazer DG, editors. Genes, Behavior, and the Social Environment: Moving Beyond the Nature/Nurture Debate. Washington (DC): National Academies Press (US); 2006. 3, Genetics and Health. Available from: https://www.ncbi.nlm.nih.gov/books/NBK19932/

Chen X, He Y, Lu F. Autophagy in stem cell biology: a perspective on stem cell self-renewal and differentiation. *Stem Cells Int.* 2018;2018:9131397. Published 2018 Jan 21. doi:10.1155/2018/9131397

Bergmann A, Steller H. Apoptosis, stem cells, and tissue regeneration. *Sci Signal.* 2010;3(145):re8. Published 2010 Oct 26. doi:10.1126/scisignal.3145re8

Alberts B, Johnson A, Lewis J, et al. Molecular Biology of the Cell. 4th edition. New York: Garland Science; 2002.

Ahmed AS, Sheng MH, Wasnik S, Baylink DJ, Lau KW. Effect of aging on stem cells. *World J Exp Med*. 2017;7(1):1–10. Published 2017 Feb 20. doi:10.5493/wjem.v7.i1.1

Kosan C, Heidel FH, Godmann M, Bierhoff H. Epigenetic erosion in adult stem cells: drivers and passengers of aging. *Cells*. 2018;7(12):237. Published 2018 Nov 29. doi:10.3390/cells7120237

Part 2

Quench

Jéquier E[1], Constant F. Water as an essential nutrient: the physiological basis of hydration. *Eur J Clin Nitr*. 2010;64(2):115-23. Epub 2009 Sep 2. doi:10.1038/ejn.2009.111

Riebl SK, Davy BM. The hydration equation: update on water balance and cognitive performance. *ACSMs Health Fit J*. 2013;17(6):21–28. doi:10.1249/FIT.0b013e3182a9570f

Environmental Working Group. "State of American Drinking Water." EWG.org.

https://www.ewg.org/tapwater/

Popkin BM, D'Anci KE, Rosenberg IH. Water, hydration, and health. *Nutr Rev*. 2010;68(8):439–458. doi:10.1111/j.1753-4887.2010.00304.x

McKiernan F, Houchins JA, Mattes RD. Relationships between human thirst, hunger, drinking, and feeding. *Physiol Behav*. 2008;94(5):700–708. doi:10.1016/j.physbeh.2008.04.007

Charfen, Alex. "Take the Natural Thirst Challenge." getthirstynow.com.

https://getthirstynow.com/natural-
thirst?_ga=2.19228472.1682930195.1551987596-
1205743360.1551987596

Breathe

Zelano C, Jiang H, Zhou G, Arora N, Scheule S, Rosenow J,
Gottfried J. Nasal respiration entrains human limbic oscillations
and modulates cognitive function. *Journal of Neuroscience.*
2016;36(49)12448-12467. Published 2016 Dec 7.
Doi:10.1523/jneurosci.2586-16.2016

Tharion E1, Samuel P, Rajalakshmi R, Gnanasenthil
G, Subramanian RK. Influence of deep breathing exercise on
spontaneous respiratory rate and heart rate variability: a
randomised controlled trial in healthy subjects. *Indian J Physiol
Pharmacol.* 2012;56(1)80-7. Published 2012 Jan-Mar.

Gerritsen RJS[1,2], Band GPH[1,2]. Breath of Life:
The respiratory vagal stimulation model of contemplative activity.
Front Hum Neurosci. 2018:12:397. Published 2018 Oct 9.
doi:10.3389/fnhum.2018.00397. eCollection 2018.

Chang RB, Strochlic DE, Williams EK, Umans BD, Liberles SD.
Vagal sensory neuron subtypes that differentially control
breathing. *Cell.* 2015;161(3):622–633.
doi:10.1016/j.cell.2015.03.022

Sharma G, Goodwin J. Effect of aging on respiratory system
physiology and immunology. *Clin Interv Aging.* 2006;1(3):253–260.

Varga S[1], Heck DH[2]. Rhythms of the body, rhythms of the brain:
Respiration, neural oscillations, and embodied cognition. *Conscious
Cogn.* 2017;56:77-90. Published 2017 Nov.
doi:10.1016/j.concog.2017.09.008

Heck DH, McAfee SS, Liu Y, et al. Breathing as a fundamental
rhythm of brain function. *Front Neural Circuits.* 2017;10:115.
Published 2017 Jan 12. doi:10.3389/fncir.2016.00115

Bonora M, Patergnani S, Rimessi A, et al. ATP synthesis and storage. *Purinergic Signal.* 2012;8(3):343–357. doi:10.1007/s11302-012-9305-8

Hamanaka R, Mutlu G. Particulate matter air polution: effects on the cardiovascular system. *Front Endocrinol (Lausanne).* 2018;9:680. Published online 2018 Nov 16. Doi:10.3389/fendo.2018.00680

Kilian J, Kitazawa M. The emerging risk of exposure to air pollution on cognitive decline and Alzheimer's disease - Evidence from epidemiological and animal studies. *Biomed J.* 2018;41(3):141–162. doi:10.1016/j.bj.2018.06.001

Zelano C, Jiang H, Zhou G, et al. Nasal respiration entrains human limbic oscillations and modulates cognitive function. *J Neurosci.* 2016;36(49):12448–12467. doi:10.1523/JNEUROSCI.2586-16.2016

American Lung Association. "Breathing Exercises." Lung.org.

https://www.lung.org/lung-health-and-diseases/protecting-your-lungs/breathing-exercises.html

Nourish

Schwalfenberg GK. The alkaline diet: is there evidence that an alkaline pH diet benefits health?. *J Environ Public Health.* 2012;2012:727630. doi:10.1155/2012/727630

Chung SM, Moon JS, Yoon JS, Won KC, Lee HW. Low urine pH affects the development of metabolic syndrome, associative with the increase of dyslipidemia and dysglycemia: Nationwide cross-sectional study (KNHANES 2013-2015) and a single-center retrospective cohort study. *PLoS One.* 2018;13(8):e0202757. Published 2018 Aug 24. doi:10.1371/journal.pone.0202757

Shimodaira M, Okaniwa S, Nakayama T. Fasting Single-Spot Urine pH Is Associated with Metabolic Syndrome in the Japanese Population. *Med Princ Pract.* 2017;26(5):433–437. doi:10.1159/000481624

Javadov S. The calcium-ROS-pH triangle and mitochondrial permeability transition: challenges to mimic cardiac ischemia-reperfusion. *Front Physiol.* 2015;6:83. Published 2015 Mar 18. doi:10.3389/fphys.2015.00083

Selivanov VA, Zeak JA, Roca J, Cascante M, Trucco M, Votyakova TV. The role of external and matrix pH in mitochondrial reactive oxygen species generation. *J Biol Chem.* 2008;283(43):29292–29300. doi:10.1074/jbc.M801019200

Sebastian A1, Cordain L2, Frassetto L3, Banerjee T4, Morris RC5. Postulating the major environmental condition resulting in the expression of essential hypertension and its associated cardiovascular diseases: Dietary imprudence in daily selection of foods in respect of their potassium and sodium content resulting in oxidative stress-induced dysfunction of the vascular endothelium, vascular smooth muscle, and perivascular tissues. Med Hypotheses. 2018;119:110-119. Epub 2018 Aug 6. Doi:10.1016/jmehy.2018.08.001

Singh Y, Zhou Y, Zhang S, Abdelazeem K, N, M, Elvira B, Salker M, S, Lang F. Enhanced reactive oxygen species production, acidic cytosolic pH and upregulated Na^+/H^+ exchanger (NHE) in dicer deficient $CD4^+$ T cells. *Cell Physiol Biochem.* 2017;42:1377-1389. Epub 2017 Jul 14. doi:10.1159/000479201

Alguacil J, Kogevinas M, Silverman DT, et al. Urinary pH, cigarette smoking and bladder cancer risk. *Carcinogenesis.* 2011;32(6):843–847. doi:10.1093/carcin/bgr048

Jan A^1, Azam M^2, et al. Heavy metals and human health: mechanistic insight into toxicity and counter defense system of antioxidants. *Int J Mol Sci.* 2015;16(12):29592-29630. Published online 2015 Dec 10. Doi:10.3390/ijms161226183

Sebastian A^1, Frassetto LA, Sellmeyer DE, Merriam RL, Morris RC Jr. Estimation of the net acid load of the diet of ancestral preagricultural Homo sapiens and their hominid ancestors. *Am J*

Clin Nutr. 2002;76(6):1308-16. Published 2002 Dec 1.
doi:10.1093/ajcn/76.6.1308

Remer T, Manz F. Potential renal acid load of foods and its influence on urine pH. J Am Diet Assoc. 1995;(7):791-797. Published 1995 Jul. doi:10.1016/S0002-8223(95)00219-7

Pizzorno J[1], Frassetto LA, Katzinger J. Diet-induced acidosis: is it real and clinically relevant? *B J Nutr.* 2010;103(8):1185-94. Epub 2009 Dec 15. doi:10.1017/S0007114509993047

Park SK, Tucker KL, O'Neill MS, et al. Fruit, vegetable, and fish consumption and heart rate variability: the Veterans Administration Normative Aging Study. *Am J Clin Nutr.* 2009;89(3):778–786. doi:10.3945/ajcn.2008.26849

Zen

Gidron Y, Deschepper R, De Couck M, Thayer JF, Velkeniers B. The Vagus Nerve Can Predict and Possibly Modulate Non-Communicable Chronic Diseases: Introducing a Neuroimmunological Paradigm to Public Health. *J Clin Med.* 2018;7(10):371. Published 2018 Oct 19. doi:10.3390/jcm7100371

De Couck M, Mravec B, Gidron Y. You may need the vagus nerve to understand pathophysiology and to treat diseases. *Clin. Sci.* 2012;122:323–328. Published 2012 Apr. doi:10.1042/CS20110299

McCraty R, Shaffer F. Heart Rate Variability: New Perspectives on Physiological Mechanisms, Assessment of Self-regulatory Capacity, and Health risk. *Glob Adv Health Med.* 2015;4(1):46–61. doi:10.7453/gahmj.2014.073

Veldhuis JD, Sharma A, Roelfsema F. Age-dependent and gender-dependent regulation of hypothalamic-adrenocorticotropic-adrenal axis. *Endocrinol Metab Clin North Am.* 2013;42(2):201–225. doi:10.1016/j.ecl.2013.02.002

Picard, M[a,b,c], McEwen B[d], Epel E[e], Sandi C[f]. An energetic view of stress: Focus on mitochondria. *Front Neuroendocrinol.* 2018;49:72-85. Published online 2018 Jan 12. doi:10.1016/j.yfrne.2018.01.001

McConnell PA, Froeliger B, Garland EL, Ives JC, Sforzo GA. Auditory driving of the autonomic nervous system: Listening to theta-frequency binaural beats post-exercise increases parasympathetic activation and sympathetic withdrawal. *Front Psychol.* 2014;5:1248. Published 2014 Nov 14. doi:10.3389/fpsyg.2014.01248

McConnell P, Froeliger B, Garland E, Ives J, Sforzo G. Auditory driving of the autonomic nervous system: Listening to theta-frequency binaural beats post-exercise increases parasympathetic activation and sympathetic withdrawal. *Front. Psychol.* 5:1248. doi: 10.3389/fpsyg.2014.01248

Hölzel BK, Carmody J, Vangel M, et al. Mindfulness practice leads to increases in regional brain gray matter density. *Psychiatry Res.* 2011;191(1):36–43. doi:10.1016/j.pscychresns.2010.08.006

McEwen BS. Protective and damaging effects of stress mediators. *NEJM.* 1998; 338:171-179. Published 1998 Jan 15. doi:10.1056/NEJM199801153380307

McEwen BS. Stressed or stressed out: what is the difference?. *J Psychiatry Neurosci.* 2005;30(5):315–318.

McEwen BS. Physiology and Neurobiology of Stress and Adaptation: Central Role of the Brain. *Physiological Reviews.* 2007;87(3):873-904. Published 2007 Jul 1. doi:10.1152/physrev.00041.2006

Zzzz

Besedovsky L, Lange T, Born J. Sleep and immune function. *Pflugers Arch.* 2012;463(1):121–137. doi:10.1007/s00424-011-1044-0

Kohatsu ND, Tsai R, Young T, et al. Sleep Duration and Body Mass Index in a Rural Population. *Arch Intern Med.* 2006;166(16):1701–1705. doi:10.1001/archinte.166.16.1701

Ayas N, White D, Al-Delaimy W, Manson J, et al. A Prospective Study of Self-Reported Sleep Duration and Incident Diabetes in Women. *Diabetes Care.* 2003;26(2):380-384. Published 2003 Feb. doi:10.2337/diacare.26.2.380

Cappuccio FP[1], D'Elia L, Strazzullo P, Miller MA. Quantity and quality of sleep and incidence of type 2 diabetes: a systematic review and meta-analysis. *Diabetes Care.* 2010;33(2):414-20. Epub 2009 Nov 12. doi:10.2337/dc09-1124

Lee JE[1], Yang SW[2], et al. Sleep-disordered breathing and Alzheimer's disease: A nationwide cohort study. *Psychiatry Res.* 2019; 273:624-630. Published 2019 Mar. doi:10.1016/jpsychres.2019.01.086

Patel SR[1]. Reduced sleep as an obesity risk factor. *Obes Rev.* 2009;10 Suppl 2:61-8. First published 2009 Oct 22. doi:10.1111/j.1467-789X.2009.00664.x

He Y[1,2], Cornelissen-Guillaume GG[3], He J[4], Kastin AJ[4], Harrison LM[4], Pan W[1]. Circadian rhythm of autophagy proteins in hippocampus is blunted by sleep fragmentation. *Chronobiol Int.* 2016;33(5):553-60. Epub 2016 Apr 14. doi:10.3109/07420528.2015.1137581

Fivenson EM, Lautrup S, Sun N, et al. Mitophagy in neurodegeneration and aging. *Neurochem Int.* 2017;109:202–209. doi:10.1016/j.neuint.2017.02.007

St-Onge MP[1,2,3], Zuraikat FM[4]. Reciprocal Roles of Sleep and Diet in Cardiovascular Health: a Review of Recent Evidence and a Potential Mechanism. *Curr Atheroscler Rep.* 2019;21(3):11. Published 2019 Feb 12. doi:10.1007/s11883-019-0772-z

Peracchia S, Curcio G. Exposure to video games: effects on sleep and on post-sleep cognitive abilities. A sistematic review of experimental evidences. *Sleep Sci.* 2018;11(4):302–314. doi:10.5935/1984-0063.20180046

Dworak M[1], Schierl T, Bruns T, Strüder HK. Impact of singular excessive computer game and television exposure on sleep patterns and memory performance of school-aged children. *Pediatrics.* 2007:120(5):978-85. Published 2007 Nov. doi:10.1542/peds.2007-0476

Bass J, Takahashi JS. Circadian integration of metabolism and energetics. *Science.* 2010;330(6009):1349–1354. doi:10.1126/science.1195027

McEwen BS. Physiology and Neurobiology of Stress and Adaptation: Central Role of the Brain. *Physiological Reviews.* 2007;87(3):873-904. Published 2007 Jul 1. doi:10.1152/physrev.00041.2006

Emory Woodruff Health Sciences Center. "Poor Sleep Quality Increases Inflammation, Community Study Finds." Emory.edu.

http://shared.web.emory.edu/whsc/news/releases/2010/11/poor-sleep-quality-increases-inflammation-study-finds.html

American Academy of Sleep Medicine. "CDC analysis finds low rate of prescription sleep aid use in U.S." aasm.org.

https://aasm.org/cdc-analysis-finds-low-rate-of-prescription-sleep-aid-use-in-u-s/

Gooley JJ, Chamberlain K, Smith KA, et al. Exposure to room light before bedtime suppresses melatonin onset and shortens melatonin duration in humans. *J Clin Endocrinol Metab.* 2011;96(3):E463–E472. doi:10.1210/jc.2010-2098

Li JY, Zhang K, Xu D, et al. Mitochondrial Fission Is Required for Blue Light-Induced Apoptosis and Mitophagy in Retinal Neuronal R28 Cells. *Front Mol Neurosci.* 2018;11:432. Published 2018 Nov 27. doi:10.3389/fnmol.2018.00432

Santini SJ, Cordone V, Falone S, et al. Role of Mitochondria in the Oxidative Stress Induced by Electromagnetic Fields: Focus on Reproductive Systems. *Oxid Med Cell Longev.* 2018;2018:5076271. Published 2018 Nov 8. doi:10.1155/2018/5076271

Javaheri S, Barbe F, Campos-Rodriguez F, et al. Sleep Apnea: Types, Mechanisms, and Clinical Cardiovascular Consequences. *J Am Coll Cardiol.* 2017;69(7):841–858. doi:10.1016/j.jacc.2016.11.069

Cooke, Rachel. "'Sleep should be prescribed': what those late nights out could be costing you." Theguardian.com.

https://www.theguardian.com/lifeandstyle/2017/sep/24/why-lack-of-sleep-health-worst-enemy-matthew-walker-why-we-sleep

Liu Y, Wheaton AG, Chapman DP, Cunningham TJ, Lu H, Croft JB. Prevalence of Healthy Sleep Duration among Adults — United States, 2014. MMWR Morb Mortal Wkly Rep. 2016;65:137–141. doi:10.15585/mmwr.mm6506a1

Movement

Jaslow, Ryan. "CDC: 80 percent of American adults don't get recommended exercise." Cbsnews.com.

https://www.cbsnews.com/news/cdc-80-percent-of-american-adults-dont-get-recommended-exercise/

Vijayaraghava A, Doreswamy V, Narasipur OS, Kunnavil R, Srinivasamurthy N. Effect of Yoga Practice on Levels of Inflammatory Markers After Moderate and Strenuous Exercise. *J Clin Diagn Res.* 2015;9(6):CC08–CC12. doi:10.7860/JCDR/2015/12851.6021

Racil G[1], Ben Ounis O, Hammouda O, et al. Effects of high vs. moderate exercise intensity during interval training on lipids and adiponectin levels in obese young females. *Euro J Appl Physiol.* 2013;113(10):2531-40. Epub 2013 Jul 4. doi:10.1007/s00421-013-2689-5

Racil G[1], Zouhal H[2], et al. Plyometric exercise combined with high-intensity interval training improves metabolic abnormalities in young obese females more so than interval training alone. *Appl Physiol Nutr Metab*. 2016;41(1):103-9. Epub 2015 Oct 15. doi:10.1139/apnm-2015-0384

Angadi P, Jagannathan A, Thulasi A, Kumar V, Umamaheshwar K, Raghuram N. Adherence to yoga and its resultant effects on blood glucose in Type 2 diabetes: A community-based follow-up study. *Int J Yoga*. 2017;10(1):29–36. doi:10.4103/0973-6131.186159

Neumark-Sztainer D, MacLehose RF, Watts AW, Eisenberg ME, Laska MN, Larson N. How Is the Practice of Yoga Related to Weight Status? Population-Based Findings From Project EAT-IV. *J Phys Act Health*. 2017;14(12):905–912. doi:10.1123/jpah.2016-0608

Neumark-Sztainer D, MacLehose RF, Watts AW, Pacanowski CR, Eisenberg ME. Yoga and body image: Findings from a large population-based study of young adults. *Body Image*. 2018;24:69–75. doi:10.1016/j.bodyim.2017.12.003

Watts AW, Rydell SA, Eisenberg ME, Laska MN, Neumark-Sztainer D. Yoga's potential for promoting healthy eating and physical activity behaviors among young adults: a mixed-methods study. *Int J Behav Nutr Phys Act*. 2018;15(1):42. Published 2018 May 2. doi:10.1186/s12966-018-0674-4

Viana RB, Naves JPA, Coswig VS, *et al.* Is interval training the magic bullet for fat loss? A systematic review and meta-analysis comparing moderate-intensity continuous training with high-intensity interval training (HIIT). *British Journal of Sports Medicine*. 2019;53:655-664. Epub 2019 Feb 14. doi:10.1136/bjsports-2018-099928

Baptista LC, Machado-Rodrigues AM, Martins RA. Back to basics with active lifestyles: exercise is more effective than metformin to reduce cardiovascular risk in older adults with type

2 diabetes. *Biol Sport.* 2018;35(4):363–372. doi:10.5114/biolsport.2018.78057

Cristi-Montero C, Chillón P, Labayen I, et al. Cardiometabolic risk through an integrative classification combining physical activity and sedentary behavior in European adolescents: HELENA study. *J Sport Health Sci.* 2019;8(1):55–62. doi:10.1016/j.jshs.2018.03.004

Durand MJ, Gutterman DD. Exercise and vascular function: how much is too much?. *Can J Physiol Pharmacol.* 2014;92(7):551–557. doi:10.1139/cjpp-2013-0486

Rush JW1, Deniss SG, Graham DA. Vascular nitric oxide and oxidative stress: determinants of endothelial adaptations to cardiovascular disease and to physical activity. Can J Appl Physiol. 2005;30(4):442-74. Published 2005 Aug. doi:10.1139/h05-133

Recinto C, Efthemeou T, Boffelli PT, Navalta JW. Effects of Nasal or Oral Breathing on Anaerobic Power Output and Metabolic Responses. *Int J Exerc Sci.* 2017;10(4):506–514. Published 2017 Jul 1.

Yetik-Anacak G[1], Catravas JD. Nitric oxide and the endothelium: history and impact on cardiovascular disease. *Vascul Pharmacol.* 2006;45(5):268-76. Epub 2006 Aug 17. doi:10.1016/j.vph.2006.08.002

Fleissner F, Thum T. Critical role of the nitric oxide/reactive oxygen species balance in endothelial progenitor dysfunction. *Antioxid Redox Signal.* 2011;15(4):933–948. doi:10.1089/ars.2010.3502

Pepine CJ[1]. The impact of nitric oxide in cardiovascular medicine: untapped potential utility. *Am J Med.* 2009;122(5 Suppl):S10-5. Published 2005 May. doi:10.1016/j.amjmed.2009.03.003

Erickson KI, Leckie RL, Weinstein AM. Physical activity, fitness, and gray matter volume. *Neurobiol Aging.* 2014;35 Suppl 2:S20–S28. doi:10.1016/j.neurobiolaging.2014.03.034

Joseph AM, Adhihetty PJ, Buford TW, et al. The impact of aging on mitochondrial function and biogenesis pathways in skeletal muscle of sedentary high- and low-functioning elderly individuals. *Aging Cell.* 2012;11(5):801–809. doi:10.1111/j.1474-9726.2012.00844.x

Walston JD. Sarcopenia in older adults. *Curr Opin Rheumatol.* 2012;24(6):623–627. doi:10.1097/BOR.0b013e328358d59b

MacInnis MJ, Gibala MJ. Physiological adaptations to interval training and the role of exercise intensity. *J Physiol.* 2017;595(9):2915–2930. doi:10.1113/JP273196

Purify

Singh R, Gautam N, Mishra A, Gupta R. Heavy metals and living systems: An overview. *Indian J Pharmacol.* 2011;43(3):246–253. doi:10.4103/0253-7613.81505

Singh N, Gupta VK, Kumar A, Sharma B. Synergistic Effects of Heavy Metals and Pesticides in Living Systems. *Front Chem.* 2017;5:70. Published 2017 Oct 11. doi:10.3389/fchem.2017.00070

Valko M1, Morris H, Cronin MT. Metals, toxicity and oxidative stress. Curr Med Chem. 2005;12(10):1161-208. doi:10.2174/0929867053764635

Sharma B1, Singh S2, Siddiqi NJ3. Biomedical implications of heavy metals induced imbalances in redox systems. Biomed Res Int. 2014;2014:640754. Epub 2014 Aug 12. doi:10.1155/2014/640754

Xu MY, Wang P, Sun YJ, Yang L, Wu YJ. Joint toxicity of chlorpyrifos and cadmium on the oxidative stress and mitochondrial damage in neuronal cells. *Food Chem Toxicol.* 2017;103():246-252. Epub 2017 Mar 9. doi:10.1016/j.fct.2017.03.013

Manikkam M, Tracey R, Guerrero-Bosagna C, Skinner MK. Plastics derived endocrine disruptors (BPA, DEHP and DBP) induce epigenetic transgenerational inheritance of obesity, reproductive disease and sperm epimutations. *PLoS One.* ;8(1):e55387. doi:10.1371/journal.pone.0055387

Thompson RC, Moore CJ, vom Saal FS, Swan SH. Plastics, the environment and human health: current consensus and future trends. *Philos Trans R Soc Lond B Biol Sci.* 2009;364(1526):2153–2166. doi:10.1098/rstb.2009.0053

Sathyanarayana S[1], Karr CJ, Lozano P, Brown E, Calafat AM, Liu F, Swan SH. Baby care products: possible sources of infant phthalate exposure. *Pediatrics.* 2008;121(2):e260-8. Published 2008 Feb. doi:10.1542/peds.2006-3766

Bailey DC, Todt CE, Burchfield SL, et al. Chronic exposure to a glyphosate-containing pesticide leads to mitochondrial dysfunction and increased reactive oxygen species production in Caenorhabditis elegans. *Environ Toxicol Pharmacol.* 2018;57:46–52. doi:10.1016/j.etap.2017.11.005

Samsel A, Seneff S[1]. Glyphosate, pathways to modern diseases III: Manganese, neurological diseases, and associated pathologies. *Surg Neurol Int.* 2015;6:45. Published online 2015 Mar 24. doi:10.4103/2152-7806.153876

Mao Q, Manservisi F, Panzacchi S, et al. The Ramazzini Institute 13-week pilot study on glyphosate and Roundup administered at human-equivalent dose to Sprague Dawley rats: effects on the microbiome. *Environ Health.* 2018;17(1):50. Published 2018 May 29. doi:10.1186/s12940-018-0394-x

Peitzsch M, Bloom E, Haase R, Must A, Larsson L. Remediation of mould damaged building materials--efficiency of a broad spectrum of treatments. *J Environ Monit.* 2012;14(3):908-15. Epub 2012 Jan 30. doi:10.1039/c2em10806b

Janette Hope[*]. A Review of the Mechanism of Injury and Treatment Approaches for Illness Resulting from Exposure to Water-Damaged Buildings, Mold, and Mycotoxins. *Scientific World*

Journal. 2013; 2013: 767482. Published online 2013 Apr 18. doi:10.1155/2013/767482

Agency for Toxic Substances and Disease Registry. "ATSDR's Substance Priority List." Atsdr.com.

http://www.atsdr.cdc.gov/spl/index.html

International Society for Environmentally Acquired Illness. "About Environmentally Acquired Illness." Iseai.org.

https://iseai.org

Consumer Reports. "How much arsenic is in your rice?" consumerreports.org.

https://www.consumerreports.org/cro/magazine/2015/01/how-much-arsenic-is-in-your-rice/

La Merrill M, Emond C, Kim MJ, et al. Toxicological function of adipose tissue: focus on persistent organic pollutants. *Environ Health Perspect*. 2013;121(2):162–169. doi:10.1289/ehp.1205485

Fry K, Power MC. Persistent organic pollutants and mortality in the United States, NHANES 1999-2011. *Environ Health*. 2017;16(1):105. Published 2017 Oct 10. doi:10.1186/s12940-017-0313-6

World Health Organization. "Persistent organic pollutants (POPs)." Who.int.

https://www.who.int/foodsafety/areas_work/chemical-risks/pops/en/

Duncan, David Ewing. "Chemicals Within Us." Nationalgeographic.com

https://www.nationalgeographic.com/science/health-and-human-body/human-body/chemicals-within-us/

Gratitude

Chen L, Bae SR, Battista C, et al. Positive Attitude Toward Math Supports Early Academic Success: Behavioral Evidence and Neurocognitive Mechanisms. *Psychol Sci.* 2018;29(3):390–402. doi:10.1177/0956797617735528

Jan YN, Jan LY. Branching out: mechanisms of dendritic arborization [published correction appears in Nat Rev Neurosci. 2010 Jun;11(6):449]. *Nat Rev Neurosci.* 2010;11(5):316–328. doi:10.1038/nrn2836

Young, Karen. "What You Focus On Is What Becomes Powerful – Why Your Thoughts and Feelings Matter." Heysigmund.com.

https://www.heysigmund.com/why-what-you-focus-on-is-what-becomes-powerful-why-your-thoughts-and-feelings-matter/

Owen L, Sunram-Lea SI. Metabolic agents that enhance ATP can improve cognitive functioning: a review of the evidence for glucose, oxygen, pyruvate, creatine, and L-carnitine. *Nutrients.* 2011;3(8):735–755. Epub 2011 Aug 10. doi:10.3390/nu3080735

Kleim JA1, Jones TA. Principles of experience-dependent neural plasticity: implications for rehabilitation after brain damage. J Speech Lang Hear Res. 2008;51(1):S225-39. Published 2008 Feb. doi:10.1044/1092-4388(2008/018)

Picard, Martin, et al. A Mitochondrial Health Index Sensitive to Mood and Caregiving Stress. *Biological Psychology.* 2018;84(1):9-17. Published 2018 Jul 1. doi:10.1016/j.biopsych.2018.01.012

Watson, Rita. "Gratitude Sparks Oxytocin and Love: Study Points to CD38." Psychologytoday.com.

https://www.psychologytoday.com/us/blog/love-and-gratitude/201402/gratitude-sparks-oxytocin-and-love-study-points-cd38

Korb, Alex. "The Grateful Brain: The neuroscience of giving thanks." Psychologytoday.com.

https://www.psychologytoday.com/us/blog/prefrontal-nudity/201211/the-grateful-brain

Morin, Amy. "7 Scientifically Proven Benefits Of Gratitude That Will Motivate You To Give Thanks Year-Round." Forbes.com.

https://www.forbes.com/sites/amymorin/2014/11/23/7-scientifically-proven-benefits-of-gratitude-that-will-motivate-you-to-give-thanks-year-round/#6061ebe9183c.

Ducharme, Jamie. "7 Surprising Health Benefits of Gratitude." Time.com.

http://time.com/5026174/health-benefits-of-gratitude/

McCraty R[1], Barrios-Choplin B, Rozman D, Atkinson M, Watkins AD. The impact of a new emotional self-management program on stress, emotions, heart rate variability, DHEA and cortisol. *Integr Physiol Behav Sci*. 1998;33(2):151-70. Published 1998 Apr.

Kini P[1], Wong J[1], McInnis S[1], Gabana N[1], Brown JW[2]. The effects of gratitude expression on neural activity. *Neuroimage*. 2016;128:1-10. Epub 2015 Dec 30. doi:10.1016/j.neuroimage.2015.12.040

Algoe S, Way B. Evidence for a role of the oxytocin system, indexed by genetic variation in *CD38*, in the social bonding effects of expressed gratitude. *Social Cognitive and Affective Neuroscience*. 2014;9(12):1855–1861. Published 2014 Jan 31. doi:10.1093/scan/nst182

Zahn R, Moll J, Paiva M, et al. The neural basis of human social values: evidence from functional MRI. *Cereb Cortex*. 2009;19(2):276–283. doi:10.1093/cercor/bhn080

Part 3

Olshansky S, Passaro D, et al. A Potential Decline in Life Expectancy in the United States in the 21st Century. *N Engl J*

Med. 2005;352:1138-1145. Published 2005 Mar 17. doi:10.1056/NEJMsr043743

Puska P, Vartiainen E, Tuomilehto J, Salomaa V, Nissinen A. Changes in premature deaths in Finland: successful long-term prevention of cardiovascular diseases. *Bull World Health Organ.* 1998;76(4):419–425.

Crinnion, Walter. *Clean, Green, and Lean: Get Rid of the Toxins That Make You Fat.* Hoboken, NJ: John Wiley, 2010.

Made in USA - Kendallville, IN
1054254_9781733129909
03.18.2020.0759